Authentic Voices, Authentic Singing:

A Multicultural Approach to Vocal Music Therapy

Sylka Uhlig

Barcelona Publishers

Authentic Voices—Authentic Singing:
A Multicultural Approach to Vocal Music Therapy

ISBN 1-891278-44-4

13 Digit ISBN 978-1-891278-44-4

2 4 6 8 9 7 5 3 1

Distributed throughout the world by:

Barcelona Publishers
4 White Brook Road
Gilsum NH 03448
Tel: 603-357-0236 Fax: 603-357-2073
Website: www.barcelonapublishers.com
SAN 298-6299

...SING

BECAUSE THIS IS A FOOD

OUR STARVING WORLD

NEEDS.

HAFIZ

(Persian poet and Sufi master, 1320-1389)

TABLE OF CONTENTS

Acknowledgements	vii
Foreword	ix
Introduction	xi
Part A: Authentic Voices	1
Chapter I	1
Professional Voices	1
Effective Voices	2
Responsible Voices	5
The Symbolic Voice — A Case Example	8
Chapter II	15
Primal Voices	15
Natural Voices	16
Shadowed Voices	18
The Isolated Voice — A Case Example	22
Chapter III	27
Acoustic Symbols	27
Maternal Voices	29
Primitive Voices	32
The Excited Voice — A Case Example	36
Chapter IV	43
Cultural Voices	43
Linguistic Voices	46
My Multicultural Voice	49
The Foreign Voice — A Case Example	52
Chapter V	57
Spiritual Voices	57
Trance Voices	61
My Transcending Voice	65
The Grieving Voice — A Case Example	67
Chapter VI	75
Neurological Voices	75
Vibrating Voices	80
Soothing Voices	82
The Silent Voice — A Case Example	84
Chapter VII	89
Methodical Voices	89
Personal Voices	90
Vocal Interventions	92
The Painful Voice — A Case Example	95

Intermezzo 101

Part B: Authentic Singing 105
Chapter VIII 107
Primitive Singing 107
Productive Singing 109
Ritualistic Singing 110
Female Singing 113
Chapter IX 119
Middle Eastern—Kurdish Singing 119
Improvisational Singing 121
Spiritual Singing 126
Islamic "Singing" 128
Chapter X 133
Native American Navajo Singing 133
Survival Singing 136
Healing Songs 139
Harmonious Singing 144
Chapter XI 147
Cultivated Singing 147
European Singing 153
Perfectionist Singing 155
Western Singing 156
Part C: Singing Practice 161
Chapter XII 163
Singing: A Personal and Professional Need 163
A Time to Sing 165
Partner Work 168
Multicultural Approach 169
Conclusion 173
Bibliography and Discography of Music of Native Cultures 175
Reprise 179
Information about Voice Workshops and Music Therapy 181
References 183
Appendix A: Kurdish Scales 191
Appendix B: Indigenous Songs 193
Appendix C: Vibration of Human Vowel 197

ACKNOWLEDGMENTS

This book is dedicated to all voices uttering sound; especially to the voice of my mother, the first authentic voice that comforted me.

My thanks to those who passionately stimulated, helped and supported me during the intense times of my studies, work, internships, travels, writings and the process of growing personally and professionally. Especially I thank all my clients I have worked with as well as my teachers, colleagues and friends. Thanks to Marianne Breuer and Ms. Börner (East-Germany), Rene Veen and Hans Storm (Netherlands), Ed van Renswouw (Netherlands), Navah Tehilla (Israel/Netherlands), Gulten Uralli (Turkey), Lisa Sokolov (USA), Barbara Hesser (USA), Diane Austin (USA), Alan Turry (USA), Ken Aigen (USA), Annette Cramer (Germany), Arthur Robbins (USA), Saskia Noordhoek Hegt (USA/Netherlands), Sabri Ateş (USA/Turkey), Heartsong Inc. (USA), staff members of P.S. 4K (USA), Susan Berkowitz (USA), John-Michael Dumais (USA) and Christoph Bouthillier (Netherlands).

Particular thanks to Kate Richards Geller, MA, MT-BC (USA) who helped my writings to become readable, understandable English and who became my collaborator and, as "voice comrade," encouraged and united with me to stay focused on the specialization of the voice. Kate Richards Geller, MA, MT-BC songwriter and music therapist, private practice, co-author of this book and co-leader of Voice workshops. SingforYourself@yahoo.com and www.TouchingVoices.com.

Special thanks to Gary Ansdell (UK) who guided and supervised my process of writing through the years and enthusiastically encouraged me not to give up. Dr. Gary Ansdell, Head of Research at Nordoff-Robbins Music Therapy Centre in London 2 Lissenden Gardens, London NW5 1PP, UK, admin@nordoff-robbins.org.uk.

Special thanks to Benedikte B. Scheiby (USA), whose amazing professional and personal supportive presence I received as student, friend and colleague. Benedikte B. Scheiby, MA, MMEd, DPMT, CMT, Assistant Director of Music Therapy at Beth Abraham Health Services, New York; clinical Adjunct Assistant Professor at the Graduate Music Therapy Program at New York University, Director of a postgraduate Training Institute in Analytical Music Therapy. BenedikteS@aol.com.

Special thanks to Joanne Loewy (USA) who peer reviewed my book and helped with professional suggestions. Dr. Joanne Loewy, DA, MT-BC, faculty member at Hahnemann University Philadelphia, instituted the Armstrong Music Therapy Program at Beth Israel Medical Center New York, edited three books– Music Therapy in Pain, NICU and in Grief and Trauma. JLoewy@bethisraelny.org.

And last but not least Nuri Akgül (USA/Turkey), whose love and powerful encouragement was with me, and without whom all this would not be possible.

FOREWORD

WHY DO WE SING?
Gary Ansdell

After nearly twenty years of working as a music therapist I'm still regularly surprised and humbled by what happens between people and music. But I'm also fairly sure about a few things now. One of these is simply that singing is often the goal to which music therapy is aiming. Or, to put it another way, what our clients really want and need to do is to sing. Even this is not quite right perhaps, since this "falling into singing" hardly seems a voluntary choice but something which just has to happen. I've seen this repeatedly in my own clinical sessions with adults or children, but also when supervising other music therapists' work, or when researching colleagues' work. I've also noticed that when music therapists present case narratives of the therapeutic process with a client often the climax of their story is when the client sings. This is really the moment when music therapy happens. And probably most of you, like me, have experienced people coming up to you after a music therapy talk and saying "All my life I've wanted to sing like that person you talked about – but the music teacher at school told me not to because of my bad voice, and I've not sung since!" One such woman was in her late 80s, and her need to sing was as strong as ever – and the frustration and sadness that accompanied this need was as important as anything else about her.

Why then do people need or want to sing? This seemingly simple question takes us (not unexpectedly given what I've already said in the first paragraph) quickly down into fundamental and existential questions about our being in the world (with ourselves, with others). It can lead to some seemingly paradoxical questions. Recently I was writing up a case study of a young man I worked with for a year in a psychiatric unit. He was in a horrible crisis in his life, overwhelmed by a dual neurological and psychiatric illness, unable to connect with family, fellow patients or staff. He often seemed half dead, took to his bed in what his psychiatrist called a 'blanket protest' against the sheer unjustness of his situation, often intoning to himself "I want to die". It sounds grim doesn't it? And yet, after a few weeks of us developing a musical relationship this man burst into song. And this song was full, loud, joyous - quite opposite to how he habitually was outside of music. He sang Beatles songs (fixating upon Let it Be with the all-too-true line for him "When I find myself in times of trouble"). But he also improvised Blues singing, and in these performances became a vibrant Blues singer (much more than I ever became a Blues pianist!). A very simple question formulated itself as I wrote this case study: Why does a man who wants to die also want to sing?

So whilst the phenomenon of singing can seem so direct, simple, natural and human, that it feels unnecessary to interrogate it with questions and theories, it's also clear from examples like this that it can warrant a depth of thinking that can tackle the magnitude of its paradoxes. Music therapy in particular seems to be able to reveal singing's paradoxes: how it seems so physical and yet mirrors the psyche and spirit so unfailingly; how it seems so individual and yet is also so culturally mediated; how it seems both an expression of identity and a medium for the communal; how (as in the example above) it can paradoxically channel eros when thanatos seems to hold sway in the psyche.

Within the current music therapy literature, however, you will have found surprisingly little sustained and systematic thinking about this complex phenomenon of singing in relation to music therapy practice. As I said earlier, you will find the literature peppered with references to the importance of singing, but to my knowledge there has been up to now no substantial monograph about singing and music therapy.

I'm delighted then that this situation is now amended with Sylka Uhlig's book. This timely and thorough work is at first look a comprehensive synthesis of interdisciplinary perspectives on many of the paradoxical aspects of singing I mentioned earlier: the physiological, psychological, social, cultural and political. This in itself would be useful to the music therapist. But much more importantly it weaves these perspectives into a moving and personal narrative of Sylka's own journey with her voice: which is also a physical, psychological, cultural, social and political story. Her own life's journey is a remarkable one – from her upbringing in the former GDR to her dedicated and varied practice as a music therapist in many clinical areas in Europe and the USA. Sylka and her relationship with singing is the golden thread that ties together the various material of this book. Her voice has been her guide, and she shows movingly how she has been able to use her trust in the 'truth of the voice' to help children and adults in challenging situations in their own lives.

Importantly, this is no sentimental narrative, as Sylka gets us to think about all the dimensions of voice and singing that make a music therapist's professional guidance reflexive and helpful. It adds to the growing music therapy literature to take the cultural and social mediation of musical communication seriously.

Why do we sing? Read this book and begin to appreciate the full complexity behind this question!

INTRODUCTION

There is something magical that happens when people are singing; I have witnessed this all my life. And specifically it caught my attention at the Ninth World Congress of Music Therapy in 1999 in Washington, DC (USA) where various presentations extolled that magical vocal expression. Music therapists around the world offered fascinating case studies but there was no exclusive approach of the voice as the primal healing instrument of every human being in every culture. I could not forget my surprise and disappointment about it and so I decided to research the topic. While I developed my own vocal methodical approach as found in this book, other music therapists who had experienced the same, used their vocal cords as they gathered to speak out about the importance of the voice.

If singing seems magical it is because we have lost touch with our natural voice and its potential to heal and profoundly affect on us. Maybe we do not understand its effect anymore and because of this we call it magical or spiritual. Maybe we are frightened of using our most intimate instrument and learning about its responsibilities. Maybe we do not know how to sing, or we are scared that we cannot sing.

Singing has never been truly magical or scary for me; it has been concrete. I have practiced singing in a variety of forms: as an innocent child; as an animated singer in music groups and bands; as a classical singer trying to be perfect in opera; as a reflecting singer, mirroring my own personality; and as an observing and singing therapist for and with my clients. Singing has not been carefree every time but repeatedly it has let me feel delighted, thrilled, ecstatic, jubilant, joyful, funny or just more sombre, broken-hearted, mournful and grief-stricken, primally touching me. Time and again when I have sung, chanted, or simply made sounds with my voice, I have gotten in touch with my unwitting sensibilities and ideas. Oftentimes it helped me directly to vent, recognize or cope with my senses, irritations and impressions, even when it sometimes confused me more initially.

During the time I sang as a child, somewhere I unconsciously sensed the sovereignty of my personal appearance. Growing up singing innocently in the suppressed society of East Germany, the former GDR, I was faced with having two lives. Outside of the house I was not allowed to voice what I thought; inside of the house I could sing, talk, and laugh, which helped me free up many of the annoyances or disillusions I carried home and safely create a little ritual.

For the duration of my technical, classical training behind the Berlin Wall, I experienced my singing as cultivated: the magnificence of making sounds was personally empowering but at the same time frustrating because my inner tension limited the sound. Through intense vocal work, I was trained to sing perfectly and beautifully but not freely. The political and personal limitations around me did not permit me to free up my voice. Moving from Alto to Mezzo Soprano, following the strict exercises for it, I struggled to sing high tones, but I never reached them because I was a prisoner of myself. But I gradually learned to send vocal, verbal messages out. I experienced finding a voice to emit my thoughts and feelings, my deliberations and sentiments, to be politically and personally active through songs.

Years later when living in the free Netherlands, my spirit demanded even more freedom from restrictions. I screamed in a pop music band and seriously damaged my vocal cords. Recovering from this and getting mature, I searched for deeper forms and expressions of freedom. I experimented with ways my voice could vibrate naturally through my whole body. I understood that I had cells and muscles, which could sensitively shake when I sang. Through bodywork and voicework I surprised myself with sounds I did not know that I could make. I met bizarre sounds coming out of me: infantile, angelic and animalistic sounds and those beautiful high ones! Amazed or embarrassed, I discovered all of them as a kind of mirror of my authentic Self.

Through work in hospitals and schools in the Netherlands, Turkey and the USA, I had discovered that adults and children were able to make beautiful, unusual, bizarre or socially unacceptable sounds like mine. I came to think of them as sending out acoustic symbols–the most spontaneous form of vocal human expression for pain, anger, grief or happiness (Chapter III). Through this and experiences over several years of travel, study, art, professional curiosity, personal communications, and many weird and wonderful musical forms, I started to pick out authentic sounds and cultural voices. Authentic means, in this context, *not imitated*; it means the original, primary form of vocal sound. Whether in languages or primitive songs, I uncovered many vocal expressions underscoring the similarities rather than the differences between human beings. I also personally experienced trance moments through singing while I was engaged in simple ritualistic forms.

The depth of all of these vocalizations and the knowledge I had collected through the years of study allowed me to consider that magic and spirituality were simply ways of discovering deeper levels of consciousness. Magic and spirituality were not strange words anymore, but perceptible in my own body and tangible for me personally through my voice.

Through the years I had been intuitively applying some of these expressive vocal forms in therapy in combination with psychotherapeutic approaches. Through the sound of my voice, I had been comforting or matching the need of many clients, even when it was only a shared sigh between two human voices. I also had unconsciously missed many valuable authentic sounds of my clients and became aware of their fear of making or receiving vocal sounds. The more I realized that, the more I opened my ears for any sound like sighing, crying, screaming, groaning, humming or singing and began to understand them as important authentic symbols of human expression. I also really valued the screaming voice of a woman which saved my own life during a car accident. Gradually, I was persuaded that the original use of authentic vocal material should become a significant part of my therapy practice and personal life.

In this book I present an eclectic selection of authentic uses of the voice to highlight its virtuosity, its healing potency and its importance to human well-being. Authentic voices can produce numerous sounds out of their emotional energy and help a person build a united personality and find one's voice. Authentic means not imitated; it means reliable, trustworthy, genuine; the original, primary use. The term "primitive song" or "primal aria"–used in an anthropologic or therapeutic sense–means nothing about the quality of the vocal music but purely the natural, authentic source: coming from the first, original, earliest kind of existence. Authentic voices carry acoustic symbols as archetypes of human expression. We can work with them as authentic symbols of unique personalities and we can value them in authentic singing in cultural perspective. This is not only pertinent in vocal or verbal therapy for our clients but also for ourselves. The music or creative art therapist, psychotherapist, teacher, singer or actor who is using his/her voice in therapy or education ought to know and experience the voice for him/herself as a primary instrument for analytic assessment, treatment or training.

Part A of this book starts with my music therapy case studies, sharing my thoughts, techniques and methods about the importance of authentic vocal material. Part B of this book is centered on traditional forms of singing in cultural perspective. From different places around the world I found common forms with which human beings express, help and heal themselves and each other through authentic singing. The commonalities of long-established and my own contemporary use portray for me the power and effect of the voice as therapeuticum[1]; incorporating primal, traditional, ritualistic, collective, cultural, theoretical, and neurological voices into methodical professionalism. In Part C of the book, describing the voice training I offer together with Kate Richards Geller, I present our workshop structure with techniques for approaching authentic voices and authentic singing as personal and professional need.

It is my hope with this book that we can learn to recognize, understand, analyze and treat vocal sounds as authentic acoustic symbols of human beings. In an analytical categorization of emotional, relational, cognitive, physical,

1. Therapeuticum: with (the effect of) healing, from the Greek terms: 'therapeia' healing and 'cum' with.

aesthetic, spiritual and technical aspects (Chapter VII), I have collected and structured my personal knowledge and experiences into a methodology. I hope that these "methodical voices" will be easily accessible to others. I also want to mention that it is possible to read over Part B, the multicultural information, and to move to Part C–another practical methodical training. While the information contained in this book is especially pertinent to the profession of the music therapist, it is also for psychotherapists, creative arts therapists, teachers, singers, actors and others who use their voice in their profession or anyone who wants to learn more about the voice. In this book, I leave out singing practices and vocal anatomy in the classical, technical sense. I also do not explain music therapy or its many variations. I recommend reading the countless books available about both voice instruction and music therapy literature[2] to support a deeper understanding of my writing. I hope that the information in this book will inspire readers to vocally express themselves more frequently for both personal pleasure and professional development. We all have the capacity to voice our most personal melodies, individual and social; it is a heritage that we have lost touch with. And we have so much to learn from different cultures and from our children, who are still carrying this innocent heritage in daily life.

---

2. See Chapter VII for more information about voice. Read Diane Austin, voice pioneer in music therapy, like Annette Cramer and Sabine Rittner, or Kristin Linklater and Paul Newham, voice pioneers in theater. For more information about music therapy, read Kenneth Bruscia's *Case Studies in Music Therapy*; or contact AMTA, the American Music Therapy Association, or WFMT, the World Federation of Music Therapy.

PART A

AUTHENTIC VOICES

Chapter I

This chapter defines the need for more attention, both in and outside the field of Music Therapy, about voice and its impact for everyone. In the *Professional Voices* section I describe the demands of a boy to be sung to in the context of professional acknowledgement of expressed needs. In *Effective Voices* I consider the effect of the voice as primary instrument for contact and communication, especially in its emotional, relational, cognitive, physical, aesthetic, spiritual and technical aspects (e.g., research on the comforting or frightening sounds of doctors reveal amazing points about the voice's effect). In *Responsible Voices* I acknowledge, together with Diane Austin and Benedikte Scheiby, the potential of the therapeutic voice as 'tool of navigation' in intensive trauma work. In *The Symbolic Voice* I review aspects of transference and countertransference through therapeutic singing with a multiple personality in psychiatric setting.

PROFESSIONAL VOICES

"You have to sing!" the 7-year-old boy dictatorially told me while I was playing piano during the music therapy session. "Why?" I asked him. "Because you have to sing 'Marcel plays the xylophone,' you have to sing for me," he answered seriously. Marcel was a small emotionally disturbed boy who had severe panic attacks and aggressive acting-out behavior, but was cognitively high functioning. He attended the school for children with special needs where I was working as a music therapist. His distractive behavior often disturbed his own concentration level as well as others' and he often used force to express his desires. His acting out was partly a reaction to his emotional insecurity, originating from home and school problems. His father temporarily left the family and Marcel seemed to be extremely attached to him and could not easily cope with his feelings of confusion. In nearly every session Marcel would hit instruments extremely hard, often the big drums, and tried to destroy them. He would cry after this outburst of anger and hide himself under the table or big drum to conceal his crying. Working to explore his feeling about his father, I once started improvising a song: "Marcel is sad because he misses his daddy." In the following sessions Marcel would demand, after his angry outburst, that I sing the "song of being sad." He would recall our improvisation about his sad feelings and whenever he reached the moment of confusion, after his rage, he would request me to sing the "song of being sad."

The above example of Marcel's acknowledgment of his need to hear my singing voice is typical, but he still surprised me each time he would order me to sing or stop singing. I believe that in the field of music therapy there is a lack of that attention given to the voice and to the essential human need it fulfils. The voice is used in nearly every session by both the client and the therapist, with little or no awareness and knowledge about its effect. The impact and effect of the voice can be to intensify or prevent self-harm in the client, which is why the therapist must learn as much as possible about his/her own instrument.

EFFECTIVE VOICES

Singing has been extremely powerful and effective for me, both personally and professionally. The voice is my strongest functioning instrument, operating flexibly whenever I need it. For Marcel, the boy described above, singing seemed to have an equally strong effect; whether or not I was singing about him did make a big difference. Often I improvise, hum and sing during therapy, vocalizing about what and how the children are playing their instruments. I also sing together with them in vocalizations and songs. Marcel ordered me to sing mostly at those moments when my voice was silent, waiting for the next step. This boy was not satisfied with my instrumental piano accompaniment. What did this boy miss in my music? What could my words or vocal sounds offer him that was more fulfilling than my piano playing? What did I carry in my voice? What need did he distinguish from my voice? Why did he repeat this request in subsequent sessions and why did he always command me to stop or encourage me to sing?

I'd like to look a bit deeper into the relationship between our human voice and our individual needs. Thinking of this boy I want to analyse my vocal expressions, separated into different levels of life, to share some of my thoughts about their importance. Here I will use an analytical categorization of emotional, relational, cognitive, physical, aesthetic, spiritual and technical aspects (I explain these later more in depth in *Vocal Interventions*, Chapter VII). The affective (emotional) level of a human vocal expression could reflect this boy's emotional existence, being alive or present with the moods he carries reflected through my singing. On a relational level of our communicative contact, if he listened to my voice, it could make him feel nurtured or provoked. The cognitive level with the symbolic representation of what he is doing could give meaning to his play on the xylophone and to his sad feelings. On the physical level, the attunement to my body-centered vocal sound could open his sense to the vibration. The aesthetic level of appreciation and repulsion of my vocal sound could provoke him either to like or dislike my singing. The spiritual level of transcendence into levels of consciousness through my vocalization could expand parts of his reality. And on a technical level the mastery of my vocal skills could provide him with an opportunity to experience my body as a musical instrument, so that my dynamics, pitch, and vibration of tone might affect him.

I created the levels above as a means to methodically analyse vocal forms as they appear in therapy. I imagine that the desires of this boy are transformed needs contained within his levels of visceral experience. Singing can connect those levels–body, mind, spirit, and emotion–providing an integrative process of becoming whole. The voice bridges all these levels and can unite them. This understanding is essential for clients' experiences, even for a boy of seven years. But this is also fundamental for the therapist's professional health. I believe that the therapist who sings in therapy sessions could also benefit from the process of growth through the levels of developing his/her own unique voice. Our personality's wholeness, experienced through vocal integration of parts of our own life story, transforms into the maturity of an authentic voice. If a therapist is singing and playing in sessions, s/he should know his/her own, earliest, most personal and natural instrument as much or more than s/he does any other instrument.

When we play piano or guitar, we have to know our instrument: the keys or strings, sound effects, melodic and tonal sequences, chord progressions, tonal color and qualities. More awareness must be required for the voice, because there is no transmitting instrument in-between: it is pure and direct. The therapist has to know how to use his/her voice and understand its intensity. The impact and effect of the sound of the voice is determined by the quality, the colors and nuances, the ranges and its limits, tone stability, breathing techniques, as well as by knowledge about vibration and resonation, and how to be comfortable in the body. Furthermore, effective use and direct impact of the voice require knowledge about positive and negative attributes of intonation, rhythm, emotional signals, and acoustic symbols. The therapist must develop awareness, sensitivity and perception about what is being communicated, verbally and nonverbally. Aspects of transference and countertransference are important to acknowledge as part of the voice's sounding.

Voice and sound specialists tell us that the speaking and singing voices have significant value in exploring a person's relationship to him or herself. The voice reveals a person's life energy and its worth. Beaulieu (1987) uses an example about this strong impact of the sound of the voice: when a doctor comes to see a patient he has the potential to frighten him and make him more ill if his voice is not harmonious. I personally know a story of a doctor who works with her father in the same family practice. She always was surprised that her father could treat some of the most difficult patients quickly with limited treatment. While she was watching their clients entering and leaving the office, her father talked to those patients, empathically listened to them and after short time they left in a satisfied and enhanced mood. She realized that because of his calming, trustworthy, therapeutic voice, he was able to help purely with his personal life energy and attitude. The medicine that he might have given would be important, but it was his authentic voice at these moments that counted.

Another example of physician sensitivity is related by Moses (1954) to show how strongly the sound of a voice affects a person and how listening can be helpful in analysing a patient's personality and condition. An experienced doctor, he says, when receiving "urgent" night calls, can decide simply by the sound of the voice–not by the words–how soon the patient should be seen. But even the risk of being sued by a patient depends on the doctor's voice as Gladwell (2005) explains in describing the startling research projects of Levinson and Ambady. Searching for the reasons for malpractice prosecutions, Levinson, a medical researcher, found that just the conversation between doctor and client made a crucial difference. He found that doctors who spent more time explaining procedures and examinations were sued less than doctors who spent less time with patients. Ambady, a psychologist, analysed this finding further, investigating intonation, rhythm and pitch. She discovered that it was not even the content of the conversation that enabled the patient to feel positive about the treatment, but the soothing sound of the doctor's voice. Not that education, experience, medicine, knowledge or responsible behaviour are not essential, but:

> If a surgeon's voice was judged to sound dominant, the surgeon tended to be in the sued group. If the voice sounded less dominant and more concerned, the surgeon tended to be in the non-sued group (Gladwell, p. 43).

This research seems incredible and we might be perplexed about the results, but if we search our experience honestly, we can all remember those simple moments when a calming voice made all the difference.

Could this be valuable in the case I described above? The boy demanded my voice with such a dictatorial tone that I felt my voice had no choice about singing or stopping. Was my voice affecting the boy more than I was aware? Did my voice carry comfort, calm him and make him feel secure? Or did it activate, irritate and provoke something in him? I believe both aspects were present in my voice and he seemed to react accordingly, telling me, through commands to sing or stop, how he felt while receiving my voice. This boy needed to be in control and used his dictatorial tone to express this. My understanding of his vocal command afforded me the choice to play in this vocal mode or not. And of course it is this knowledge and awareness of the sound of the voice that leads one to a better understanding of our clients and ourselves as well. Intuitive judgments appear every moment when human beings communicate through their voices. Some voices are too shrill or too dreary for our ears or there are unpleasant sounds to which we are sensitively reacting. This applies not only to therapy or teaching, where we can use the voice as diagnostic tool, but also to our everyday operative functional voice as well.

RESPONSIBLE VOICES

Through my experience with adults and different forms of music therapy–the active form of singing and playing instruments and the receptive form of listening to recorded music and Guided Imagery through Music (GIM)[3]–I have learned that some clients are extremely sensitive to the sound of human singing voices. In my own practice, many clients have taught me how complicated the intimacy of the voice can be for them. Children have reacted with evident repulsion or acceptance as in the case example of Marcel. Many adults have expressed their resistance to letting in or receiving vocal sound because it can be excessively intense. They have judged vocal sounds more critically than instrumental music. They have refused to listen to recorded vocal music and could not accept the closeness of the penetration of a human voice. Others, have been so terrified by the feeling of being heard that they never opened their mouth, nor uttered any sound, not even humming or softly singing.

Possible answers for the healing as well as frightening quality of the human voice can be found in its sudden and deep, penetrating appearance. Without cognitive filtering any sound can go directly through our ears and affect our minds and bodies. Unable to protect ourselves from this intimacy, human sounds can be interpreted as an insistent vocal attack. This may cause people to reject vocal sounds if they are not connected to a safe environment and also to resist their self-healing qualities to avoid connection with themselves. This fear of intimacy of the voice needs to be softened through trustworthy therapeutic relationships where, through a kind of modern ritual, a safe space for experience and exploration can be created. This voice must also be frightening to our contemporary cultures because of its magically beneficial and human effect, an effect that contradicts the experience of disconnection in a machine age, when the integration of the voice into ritual has been severely diminished.

Most alternative healing therapies are not focused on an intense therapeutic relationship between client and therapist, and many of them are working with big groups and in workshop settings where this relationship is not feasible. I hold that in the psychotherapeutic approach, where the original roles of early parent-child relationships always emerge, intimacy and safety are

---

3. GIM: Guided Imagery through Music was developed by music therapist Helen Bonny (USA) in the 60's and is used in a variety of settings and populations.

crucial aspects, especially because of the power of the voice. Both female and male music therapists should be cognizant of the maternal and paternal impact of their feminine or masculine voices. The voice emits one's true personality; the therapist's role as good or not-good-enough mother/father is projected through his/her vocal expression and body language more than through words: here, transference and countertransference appears[4].

Diane Austin works vocally with adults in psychotherapeutic private practice music therapy. Most of her clients have 'preverbal wounds,' meaning that their trauma developed when vocabulary and syntax were not yet manifested to express the feelings about it. Austin is clear to explain about the deep access potential that the voice can evoke. The client's fear of a "projection of the vulnerable, undeveloped young part of the self" (1998, p. 315) through singing is serious; the therapist should be aware of this and create an extremely safe therapy environment. Or perhaps some clients "avoid singing unison" (singing in same pitch or octave), not ready for this kind of close relationship, and the therapist needs to sing unison because of his/her personal attachments to symbiosis.

Much is written about the need for the therapist's awareness of his/her own relationships, which are played out in contact with the client. The therapeutic relevance for this kind of sensibility is emergent in vocal relationships. The therapist's early awareness of a client's traumatic history often first appears in vocal sounds, coming from countertransference reactions. The more a therapist is able to sense his/her presence and this musical/vocal countertransference, the earlier s/he can intervene. Being responsive to the client's vocal sounds needs to occur in every session. The understanding of these personal emotional issues and knowledge about them has an immeasurable impact upon the therapist's personal and professional growth.

I believe that the vocal impact of the countertransference effect is intensely more profound than one might expect. The voice, as our earliest instrument for contact and communication, should be seen as a tool of navigation, as Scheiby (1998) calls any musical contact in music therapy. In the musical contact, the sound of the voice is accessing a pathway of intimate relationship that young children once experienced with their parents, their personal attachments and symbiosis. The therapist's voice in this intimate contact can function either as a key to healing or re-traumatizing. Scheiby warns about unconscious roles getting projected onto the therapist as well as the client: from "the seducer" to "the seduced," from "the helpless, impotently enraged

---

4. Transference, psychoanalytical: reproduction of emotions esp. those experienced in childhood toward a person other than the one toward whom they were initially experienced;
Countertransference: transference on the part of the analyst of the repressed feelings aroused by the analysand (Stein, 1966, The Random Dictionary).

victim" to "the sadistic abuser," from "the inner neglected, abused child" to the "rescuer and protector" (Scheiby, pp 234-235). It is possible that we, as therapists, are re-experiencing our own childhood traumas in the therapy with our traumatized clients and that our clients are practicing the same.

The awareness of those roles helped me better understanding my own patterns and deep-seated effect of my early relationships on my current interactions with clients. Through awareness, sensitivity and ongoing supervision where I analysed my mistakes, I became more conscious of the possibility of transforming countertransference: first, I consciously listened to my voice; second, I critically judged the sounds of my own voice as a therapist; and third, I became able to alter my vocal sounds, focusing on the needs of my client. During my vocal exploration I experienced singing with a partner and getting myself vocally mirrored. I carefully listened to my vocal recordings, analysed my role-plays and vocally improvised extensively outside of my work settings to become comfortable with my own sounds. All of these aspects, and the roles, stages, memories, and innate intensity of the voice, heightened my awareness. After years of personal experience and work, I trained myself to discover the mirrors of my vocal sounds. And I learned that a music therapist carries the responsibility of the impacts that s/he can have on clients and should be able to enter the clinical interaction with an experienced and knowledgeable voice as a tool for navigation.

There is no instrument so personal and rooted with the experience of individual life than the voice. When we sing, scream, cry and laugh, we do this with our bodies: the body is our instrument. Our instrument has been played and treated in different ways through the years by a variety of others: our mothers and fathers, teachers, friends, relatives, siblings. And everybody 'touched,' 'used' or 'played' with us–possibly with love and softness, but perhaps also with rigidity, violence or abuse. All of these influences are stored in our minds and bodies as memories. I believe that our bodies have a memory too, which is saved physiologically in our muscles and reflexes. We react as our bodies were taught to react in different situations with tension and defence, release and relaxation, fight or flight (see Chapter VI). We still can hear some of these memory traces in a person's voice. The voice tells us about one's past, memories, and life story. It is the sound of our feelings and the timbre of our life. And when a person's voice is awakened with all of these memories, we can hear the person's life story in this sound.

But some of these memories are buried deep and we cannot easily hear them. Some stories are too painful and it was safer to isolate them far from sound into silence. It was safer to forget them or to store them in the unconscious. Through using our voices we are able to stir and access some of these old memories, in our mind's and body's conscious and unconscious. We can evoke deep, painful feelings or happy joyful experiences of our childhood.

When we sing, we are using our earliest familiar instrument, and we can touch these early feelings and thoughts. We can awaken these feelings and thoughts by vibrating and resonating the cells and muscles of our instrument. We can sense the resonance of our instrument and we can reconnect to our memories through it. We can conjure up our early experiences and perhaps bring them toward conscious daily life.

We have the choice to reconnect with our memories and experiences or not. Sometimes these experiences are too painful and it is better to let them sleep in the unconscious. Sometimes painful ones arise unprovoked and need to be integrated into our daily life to make us whole and authentic. The therapist's voice in this context can function as healing or re-traumatizing, depending on the personal attachments, symbiosis and the client's symbiosis. The sound of the therapist's voice enters the space of intimate relationship that young children experienced with their parents.

The use of songs can touch these early memories too, sometimes by chance, sometimes intentionally. Both the therapist's and client's voice when singing songs can awaken the emotions around the song. They can bring forgotten or suppressed feelings back through touching old emotions or through the content of the lyrics. Singing can bring us in contact with early memories and thoughts of being lost, for example, or the memory of being shut up, the exile of 'life in silence.' But when this memory is given a sound or voice, it is invited out of the silence and the old pain of being shut up may also appear with it. This pain is big and powerful because it has been feeding the existential fear being silenced. A lot of energy was needed to keep it silenced for all these years. The silence of being shut up, of not being able to babble, to cry, to scream, to talk, to laugh, to sing, or make funny sounds as children do–this silence formed and forced the growth of an extreme personality. The therapist's voice and its knowledge about these aspects have a crucial function in the process of awakening the client's voice, and in setting safe boundaries.

THE SYMBOLIC VOICE – A CASE EXAMPLE

I remember an exceptional client I worked with for three years in the psychiatric hospital in the Netherlands. A young woman, I'll call her Bella, was suffering from a personality disorder called Multiple Personality Syndrome (MPS). She was a gifted, intelligent woman in her twenties from an educated family. The suspicion of ritualistic abuse and her accusation of early sexual abuse by her family members traumatized her from early childhood until young adult age. She was restricted to strong controls in the hospital, unable to leave the unit alone because of her tendency to run away during times of confusion. The psychotherapist advised that Bella needed to learn the difference between secure and insecure situations, and besides that to practice any positive experiences. Bella loved music, played the flute, piano and wanted to sing, but did not dare. She came to music therapy because of her interest in music and the need for positive experiences.

I first worked with her on the search for a place in the room, creating a safe island where she could feel secure. I put chairs in a corner of the room in different circles and let her determine how close I could come. For months we discovered levels of fear of distance and closeness, talking about changing her location in the room while listening to music. Our relationship circled around building elementary trust, a trust dependent on my personal and professional appearance and her ability to reject or accept me. After 6 months Bella wanted to learn how to sing and I offered technical singing instruction. When she joined the singing group of traumatized women, a frightening experience for her, she could hardly open her mouth. Quietly singing and experimenting a bit with different instruments, she developed her first sense of safety in the music group. She requested individual singing lessons from me to become more comfortable with her voice. Intensive therapy work with the voice would have forced a premature confrontation for her traumatized and obese body. I decided to start with singing lessons, focusing not on feelings about songs yet, but on how to set 'practical' boundaries.

One year later, during our individual therapy, Bella was mature enough to be able to sit close to me and conduct herself more comfortably. She brought in personal songs and asked if I could sing them for her. I started learning and singing her songs at her request with a performing and leading voice. Herein lay for me some similarity with her experience of abuse–following a leader, either the abuser or any dominant person. While I was singing her songs, she searched for the right melody, vocal timbre, and interpretation while vocalizing in the background of my sound. I verbally and vocally encouraged her to produce more sound and stronger expressions but she was not able to express herself loudly. She needed me to model sounds vocally and emotions that she had not developed herself. Using my voice both as a shelter and a tool for navigation, Bella continued her role of singing tenderly. Singing that way seemed to expand her trust between our voices: my dominant singing, expressing various emotions, seemed to create feelings of safety. She gave the impression of feeling sheltered through the range of my sounds, softly discovering affective expressions herself. Little by little she found the courage to be more connected to the melodies and contents of the songs, and her singing became lightly expressive. Bella began to sing all of the songs with a variety of voice qualities, searching for her authenticity. The fear of being heard, and the chance of punishment for taking such a risk came up when she created her own sound. She was unconscious of projecting her memories and her role of helpless victim; her inner neglected, abused child needed a rescuer, a protector. It appeared to me that she gave me that protecting role. Accepting this responsibility intensified my vigilant caution about the use of my voice. My vocal navigation skills were tested: not overwhelming her but sturdy enough to support her emotional defences, explosion or shutting down.

Following my agreement with the psychotherapist, I stayed focused on vocal techniques to avoid premature concentration on her emotions and their overwhelming effect on her. Through these techniques she felt safe and able to experiment with stronger sounds and interpretations without any direct emotional over-stimulation. Bella learned voice and breathing techniques, expanded her vocal range, and for the time being, stayed away from the exercises that might re-traumatize her. I helped her experiment with colors, nuances and limits of sound, and tone stability. I taught her about vibration and resonance, and how to sing comfortably in the body. The delicate pacing of her therapy was crucial.

When I started to look closely at the songs Bella was bringing in, I discovered that nearly all of them were children's songs. I realized that every one of these songs was a symbol for a level of her development. In collaboration with her primary psychotherapist, my team colleague, we discovered that each song corresponded to a specific age and significant moment in her life where she was abused and traumatized. She had split off these parts of her personality into silence and now she was unconsciously bringing them to music therapy. Starting with the parts she liked about herself, she brought songs about positive experiences. In a later stage she brought songs for the 'bitch' in her, as she called it.

In her verbal psychotherapy Bella was able to switch between these different personalities, giving them clear names and functions but unable to connect to them emotionally. There was an inner wisdom in her that knew that these splits needed attention and healing. It seemed that her unconsciousness was acting in a healthy way in her attempt to musically connect her different personalities.

I supportively sang Bella's songs with her while I developed a sense about their meaning, and bit by bit Bella made real contact with them. Through the lyrics she revealed more about her life stories. Verbally she shared thoughts and processed some of her experiences. But vocally we expressed the pleasure, pain, hate and fear she carried in her mind and body. She was able to laugh from discomfort, shriek with fun or stay silent with embarrassment; but crying in front of me was a significant shift because the 'little girl' in her was not allowed to cry in her childhood. I vocally mirrored, shared and comforted her authentic sounds and learned how significant it was to communicate through my voice as a form of human contact. It also opened me vocally to the various moods and age of her childlike stages, addressing the interpretation or context of the songs. I became able to sing as a child does–silly, sad or rebellious–and in the process re-awakened those parts in myself.

One by one we sang the songs, and with each I first vocally connected myself where I expected the age of the child to be until Bella could follow me. First imitating me but later, still unconscious about her suppressed developmental stages, she progressively transformed the quality of her own voice according to the role and age she chose in the songs. In one song she was strong and confident, a kind of rebel, opponent or fighter; in another she was an infant, a tiny, innocent, frightened girl that did not dare to come into the forefront. In the protection of my leading sound, experiencing more and more security, Bella started to express these roles more clearly. It took her months before she dared to shout with me during a song about her abusive environment. This unforeseen unity of our human voices created such a bond between us that she repeated that song for weeks. At other times she used a whispering, high-sounding voice to express her need for intimacy and attachment in a song. I vocally tuned into this need and incorporated her symbolic language of an infant, humming or singing to nurture her sounds.

All of the songs/ages formed important split-off parts of Bella's life and the MPS symptoms became increasingly problematic. Emotionally she was not able to connect these different parts of herself into one whole personality. In conversation at one moment, she could react as a little girl with a high voice and in the next moment as an intellectual adult with a low and controlled voice. She was not aware of these switches–this was normal for her in moments when she was out of control and felt insecure. By singing her songs, she deepened their contexts and emotional meanings, resonated with her split-off parts, and discovered them as parts of herself, parts of her body and mind. It was important to bring her personal songs out of the silence, to voice their sound, allowing her to express:

- the fearful 3-year-old singing a simple song like "Baba Black sheep"
- the angry 6-year-old uttering a fairytale song about an "Air Castle"
- the panicking girl of 8 interpreting "Do, Re, Mi"
- the mistrusting, willful teenager of 13 pressuring to "Give me my flowers"
- the developing self-esteem of a 16-year-old expressing "I am what I am"
- the intelligent, independent young woman of 19 singing a classical song by Vivaldi.

It was surprising for me to watch how intensely Bella's singing transformed into different levels of development and consciousness[5]. Expanding the sense of reality, place and time, she vibrated with one of those split-off parts of her childhood and simultaneously she was herself the adult, present here in the music therapy room.

Once Bella brought a song with two parts, the fairy and the witch, offering me the role of the adoring fairy. Realizing her progress in therapy, I decided that we would work on both roles, thinking that the role of the witch for her could be too intense. After 6 months of intensive vocal exploration and internalization of both roles, using beautiful vocalizations for the fairy and bizarre, really frightening sounds for the witch, we revealed the authenticity of our vocalization. With support of the drama therapist, using costumes and rehearsing our roles, Bella and a small group of female clients performed the story of the fairy and the witch. I performed the role of the witch in a duet with her, using such vocal authenticity that the 'little ones,' as Bella called the young split-off parts, got a bit scared. But knowing that I was the performer of the witch made her feel safe, she said. Vocally and physically triumphing over the witch in the role of the fairy, she had acted and worked her through tremendous, intense fear. We concluded this stage of therapy with a dramatic performance for a video recording of ourselves. At first it was scary for Bella to watch the video, but unexpectedly she was impressed by her own excellent performance of the fairy and of her distancing of the witch.

At the end of this process Bella suddenly gave me a song about her dead baby that had been born out of an abusive relationship. Singing a song about such a broken-hearted subject brought my tears up and, unsure if I should continue, I sought further supervision. Considering the incredible sensitivity of this issue and being hesitant myself, I worked closely with her psychotherapist. Bella and I sang that song carefully with soft and tender voices in the sessions. Touching every emotional string in our bodies during the following weeks, I vibrated vocally with Bella's pain. Realizing the importance of this subject for her, I slowly encouraged her to sing the song alone, while I guided her attunement and soothed her sorrow with my voice. For months she worked hard, stopping when tears overwhelmed her or when images snowed her under. But Bella followed the stream of her vocalizations, adjusting and regulating the pain herself: for the first time in her life she experimented with mastering her own emotions. After 4 months I felt the need for a bridge to the outside world and we

---

5. See phases of development in different psychological theories of Freud, Erikson and Piaget. All developmental stages of children are categorized in similar age groups. Bella seemed to be delayed due to her traumatic childhood experiences. If a child does not develop according to those stages, the need to express these related needs stay alive into adulthood, as Janov explains in *The Primal Scream* (see Chapter II). In Bella's case there was a need to sing young children's songs as well as to cry, scream, yell or laugh like young children do.

invited the psychotherapist to listen to her singing. While she sang shyly, caring and mourning about her own baby with a heartbreaking authentic voice, the psychotherapist wept. Being her bystander for so long, I felt relieved to carry over some of the responsibility to another witness and part of her support system. Through those songs, Bella carefully became able to express parts of herself, and looking at them, she started to connect them. The sounds she learned to make about her life story through her voice enabled her to get in touch with the anger of the abuse, to sing as an infant without danger, and to mourn about the dead. It helped Bella to integrate these parts of herself into one personality. Her pain emerged and did not subside right away, but the silence became a sound, a sound of a relieved human voice. Bella told me at the end of our three-year work relationship that the music therapy sessions were very important for "us," referring to her split-off parts, because "all of us felt safe and we were allowed to be." The different parts of her personality dared to come out in our songs. Touched by watching those parts developing a voice, little by little I saw her existential fear decreasing and my set boundaries receding.

Humbly and gradually liberated, Bella's authentic personality began to grow and her voice grew with her. This voice experienced the freedom of giving sound instead of being shut up. This voice vibrated and opened her body's resonance through singing, shouting, crying, laughing or making numerous silly sounds. She started to produce new sounds and to clean up the old frozen energy in her body. Her voice seemed to be reborn and ultimately she left the hospital, returning to music therapy on an outpatient basis. That she returned to maintain musical contact was proof of the trust that had been established both in our therapeutic relationship and in our relationship with our human voices. Saying goodbye to me, she offered as a present a song she had: giving all the parts of her personality a special voice, each singing 'thank you.' We had established an extraordinary unity and it gave me joy to help her with an application for a musical, educational program to support her future development.

> When a man is singing
> And cannot lift his voice
> And another comes and sings with him,
> Another who can lift his voice,
> Then the first will be able to lift his voice too
> That is the secret of the bone
> Between spirit and spirit.

Martin Buber, 1947, "Tales of the Hasidim"

Chapter II

In this chapter I describe the universal human vc
vehicle for expression. In Primal Voices, referenci
describe the importance, assessment and analysis of
personality. Natural Voices distinguishes the power a … voice in a natural context by comparing it with animal sounds. For instance, to cry out from happiness or danger is socially acceptable, whereas to groan, yawn, weep or scream is not always tolerated. But we need to express and accept both as I describe in Shadowed Voices, where Wolfsohn's "voice in extremis" opens this potential of bright and shadow sounds as healthy flow of our emotional energy. In The Isolated Voice, referring to Wilber's description of the 'little barbarians' in us, I consider the scream of a deprived voice as a form of therapeutic catharsis in a psychiatric setting.

PRIMAL VOICES

The human voice is our earliest, most unique and most natural instrument for primary expression and communication. The voice is also our most intimate instrument and gives us the opportunity to make contact with ourselves and our environment. The voice can be seen as a very active agent in our personal and professional relations. The voice can work for us or against us every moment, in social, work-related, or very intimate interactions. It always writes the anthology of our emotions.

Paul Newham offers the following description of the voice for physical and psychotherapeutic analysis and identification with the whole personality:

> The voice is the expression of who we are and how we feel. In the timbre of a person's voice you can hear the subtle music of feeling and thought. The ever shifting collage of emotions which we experience infiltrates the voice with tones of happiness, excitement, depression and grief. The human voice is also one way in which we preserve our identity and the voice and the psychological state of an individual mutually influence each other. The physical condition of the body is also reflected in the vitality of vocal expression: illness,

physical debilitation and habitual patterns all take their toll on the way we sound (1998, p. 24).

The voice as an active agent, a kind of representative, is always in attendance and tells us who we are and how we feel, how our physical and psychological past and present conditions are affecting us at any particular moment. The voice, as the speaker of our identity, transverses the brain and body, connects emotions and thoughts. The claim that the voice can work for you or against you carries the interesting implication that it is almost impossible to hide feelings and thoughts behind your voice; at least something of these personal expressions will be heard through talking, singing or making sound.

We know a lot about the most primitive expressions of fear, pain and anger by listening to animals. Early attempts to analyse the voice were provided by Porta, a sixteenth-century Neapolitan physician who compared animal sounds to human sounds. Porta was seeking analogies between animals and human beings by evaluating human types against certain animal types, carrying any likeness in their physiognomy to the human, and finding similarities in their respective voices. Through voice analysis, he later translated these prototypical discriminations of morphology into different types of men and culture.

NATURAL VOICES

Human and animal voices bear a close and powerful resemblance. I believe that this provides a unique insight into ancient traditions and their relationship to nature.

In early and primitive cultures, human beings were imitating the sounds of animal voices to connect themselves with their natural environment. This connection made them feel safe and powerful and also bonded them strongly with nature itself. This connection helped people survive in dangerous situations and celebrate and bond in joyful ones. The voice had the role of a crucial instrument for personal and communal expression in moments of happiness and pleasure, grief, sadness and fear as well as to protect, to warn or to invoke.

This connection between animals and human beings can be described as a process of empowerment with natural and spiritual elements. In many early cultures where animals shared daily life with humans, it was believed that nearly every natural element, object or product was empowered through the soul or spirit of a special animal or totem[6]. Their authentic meanings of empowerment

---

6. Totem: natural object or animate being to which a family or clan considers themselves closely related.

were transcribed into sounds and movements most likely to contain this spirit. To celebrate the powerful bear in a ceremony, for example, native people sang about the bear or imitated its voice. To become united with the bear's soul they contributed rituals: singing or voicing about its environment, the sun, moon, soil and water. The earth with its natural sources became sound, an acoustic symbol, and a "vital cry" as Newham calls it. The voice connected human beings strongly to nature through the sounds they made. Every aspect of life uttered a sound; every element of life was connected to sound. With their most portable instrument human beings have been able for centuries to give natural sound to everything and to any kind of condition or situation.

Today many powerful vocal expressions are going unnoticed; they are unconscious or have lost their significance as crucial and functional for living creatures. Barking dogs calling for attention, singing birds communicating messages, yelling mothers protecting their children, weeping grown-ups mourning the loss of a loved one, groaning patients or dying soldiers moaning in pain–we hear and see these expressions but most likely with no special attention.

I also personally experienced the power of the voice through a fearful moment of an accident years ago. The powerful voice of a woman called out to stop a van that had knocked me down on the street and was about to run me over. This woman's scream was like a natural siren, an instinctive connection to her environment. Like a shrieking animal to inform of present danger, this woman's scream stopped the van that was backing up and not noticing me. With her little but authentic female voice, acting in the moment, she got the driver's attention. He stopped, not knowing that I was already under his van. Her voice prevented a big disaster and I fortunately survived!

If I compare these dramatic sounds of calling, warning and mourning, I can hear common patterns of expression between human beings and animals. Also when I listen to my voice in uncontrolled, private situations–when I groan, yawn, weep and scream–I can hear my instincts before they reach my awareness. I am balancing between my instincts and intellect; often comfortable when I am in private and only now and then I am afraid that I might lose control of them in public. But I also can hear the comparison when I listen to patients who have lost their voice or their usual communication capacity. Some of them can only make instinctual sounds such as moans, groans or wails. And they are not in private but in a hospital. As a therapist I can accept their frightening sounds, thinking it reminds me of animals. The same is true with children with limited or no language skills. I have to learn to recognize, accept and to work their sounds as human. In fact, those sounds are not so unusual; the voice in its purest and simplest form is designed to express primary feelings–pain, fear, anger and joy–and most of those sounds do not sound beautiful.

The German voice pioneer and physician, Alfred Wolfsohn[7], experienced the incredible sounds of the voices of wounded and dying soldiers in the trenches during the First World War. He became horrified and fascinated by it, and surprised and shocked to hear how a human voice could utter such a sound, "a voice in extremis." After being exposed to those sounds Wolfsohn suffered terribly from aural hallucinations of the earnest screams and groans of the dying. But he also found a cure for it by actually singing out loud the sounds he had heard. Through expanding the range of his voice and remembering the impressive disturbing sounds he was exposed to in the trenches, Wolfsohn found that his voice could express a similar anthology of emotions. Wide ranges of tempers, both suffering and joyful sounds, he uttered with pleasure and curiosity. Discovering a form of personal vocal catharsis, he was able to cure his hallucinations and identified that "there exists a universal human voice of much broader circumference than has hitherto been imagined."

This 'universal human voice' has the ability to cry, laugh, scream, moan, talk, sing and much more. Based on my own experience I believe that some of these vocal expressions, such as crying, laughing and singing, are very closely linked to one another and the transition from one expression to the other is made easily, i.e. there is no existing border between them. It is possible to slide through these vocal expressions from one thought or emotion to another–from crying into singing, from laughing into crying or vice versa. For example, Sing-crying–when a sustained cry takes over a certain tonality and rhythmic structure while staying unconscious and not being manipulated–is a comforting phenomenon. It reminds me often of my own mood changes when I was a child: the natural stream of this flowing, emotional expression moved me into a simple melodic or rhythmic pattern that finally comforted me. There was no shift in between, any change of intention to sing after crying. This emotional fluidity is an identifying factor of what made me a human being; animals express their basic feelings, sensations or affections through sound, but only human beings are able to cry, laugh and sing and to combine them with other emotions.

SHADOWED VOICES

Wolfsohn experienced his own shadow, or dark side, through singing the horrifying sounds he had heard. He discovered that a singer had the capacity to penetrate deep into the depths of his own body and touch a new and unknown sound in his voice. And when he listened to it, it sounded like a voice of a stranger, a foreigner. I am acquainted with the concept that, through the voice,

7. Wolfsohn in Newham (1989).

human beings can make contact with each other through sounds and languages. But also by listening to the sounds of our voices, we get in touch with our own shadows. Following Wolfsohn, I learned that the shadow is the complement of the light and nothing can shine in the light without having a shadow. The same light/shadow principle is present for every aspect of human life.

Wolfsohn realized when he was teaching singing, that the range of his students' voices was not controlled by physiological aspects but by their psychological limitations. He stimulated them to extend their ranges, to experiment with unusual sounds, making up their own languages and discovering their voices as a mirror of their personalities. When his students made contact with their own shadows through vocalizing unusual and antisocial sounds, a kind of primitive and animal side of their personality was revealed. The shadow in the voice sounds as if it's coming from a lower level, from the instinctive and animalistic, the dangerous, unknown, uncultivated or rough part of the personality. Or it could be interpreted as the sound of a strange or foreign-speaking or -singing person: a different archetype of linguistic expression.

Wolfsohn concluded that if the voice is the true mirror of the personality and of its psyche, then the voice should express the needs of its shadow through screaming, yelling, shrieking, and clicking as the instinctive, animalistic part of the personality. And Wolfsohn's approach to singing facilitated the spontaneous emergence of an extraordinary variety of unusual sounds. These sounds had a particular meaning for each pupil, helping them tap into and relive a deeper echelon of their evolutionary past. This was a far cry from singing beautifully, Wolfsohn remarked. It was squeaking and squeezing, screaming and peeping and most significantly: it was authentic.

All of these expressions come from one and the same source of "emotional energy," as Jung called it. This emotional energy is the natural source of creativity, emotion, and unconscious imagination, and unfortunately many are often disconnected from it. Without knowing what they miss, human beings search for deeper connections, which drive them to investigate a larger connection with the cosmos through Eastern body techniques like yoga, artistic classes in music, dance, art, or spiritual forms of religion and philosophy. The human dilemma of feeling lost and isolated originated exactly from that experience of non-integration, being disconnected from natural sources. Jung describes the break-up with nature as the loss of that emotional source of energy:

> Man feels himself isolated in the cosmos, because he is no longer involved in nature and has lost his emotional 'unconscious identity' with natural phenomena. These have slowly lost their symbolic implications. . . . His contact with nature has gone, and with it has gone the profound emotional

> energy that this symbolic connection supplied (Jung, 1964, p. 95).

If I think of the voice as the biological and psychological instrument of the Self, then I am still surprised how little we know about its expressions. Somehow the fully powerful voice has been perceived as threatening, and so we have come to fear our earliest instrument. Its vast potential carries our characteristic authenticity and power, but we do not use it sufficiently. The singing and speaking voice of a person is formed through the requirements of the culture, the society and the environment. Since the shadow side of the voice does not harmonize with the requirements of a refined society, we have in our quest to "fit in" eliminated it.

There is a correspondence between civilized Western vocal expression and the stages of consciousness development. Our consciousness is limited by our civilized vocal expressions, and both mind and voice reflect our distance from natural sources. Ken Wilber (1996) pictures the stages of consciousness in a humorous way and I'd like to cite his thoughts. He says that we have a potential of 100 units of natural awareness when we are born; when we are very young, we lose 10 percent of it:

> 10 percent of [a person's] awareness is stuck at moral stage I, stuck in this little unconscious blob residing in the basement and using its 10 percent of awareness in an attempt to get the entire organism to act according to its archaic wishes and impulses and interpretations . . . by the time the self reaches adulthood, it might have lost 40 percent of its potential, as split-off or dissociated little selves, little blobs, little *hidden subjects*, and these little subjects tend to remain at the level of development that they had when they were split off. So you have these little barbarians running around in the basement. . . . [These barbarians] scream and yell and bite and claw, and since you don't even consciously know they are there, you *interpret* this interior commotion as depression, obsession, anxiety, or number of neurotic symptoms that are completely baffling (p. 154).

And these barbarians try to follow their archaic wishes and impulses in order to be natural and not moralistic. The uncultivated, instinctive voice belongs to this behavior; it is rough and wild, and as authentic as can be. Its vocal potency must be as rich as its authentic expressions of screaming or yelling, and must include the shadow sounds. If these sounds are not allowed to escape the body then they might later become the voices of depression and anxiety. So let's integrate them.

I consider that the general range of the voice has changed through the centuries from the voice-as-being to the voice-as-social-instrument. In technological societies like Western Europe and North America, and increasingly also in the big cities of third world countries, we see the same trend. And all of the possible sounds of the authentic voice-as-being are still present in their natural potential. Culture is limiting these ranges and is making the voice into a social instrument that is acceptable to society. In today's industrialized, civilized cultures with their highly technological focus, which espouses life's comforts, can we expect that the voice will–after all of these restrictions through the centuries–recover from its limitations and slowly reclaim a more natural, authentic sound? Will we be able to rediscover and re-experience the range, power and the potency of the voice for our bodies and psyche, including the shadow sounds, without becoming impolite and rough? Is it necessary to do this? And if yes, what will be the ultimate result?

Given modern man's distance from his authentic voice, it's necessary to negotiate to find a balance between the little barbarians and their social acceptance. To be effective we need to integrate instead of repress. Fighting against our shadows has not been satisfying thus far. We have the chance to get involved in this process and cultivate awareness, awakening and adopting the primitive, authentic voice as a healthy instrument for all human beings in all societies. Maybe, in this process, we can tap into the emotional energy as source of wellness. Maybe we keep searching without knowing what we are missing. But maybe we can feed our unconscious identity with nature to heal depression, anxiety, and other forms of isolation.

Independent of culture, history, gender and personality, there are universal sounds that all human beings produce. The function of the voice is the same everywhere: expression, contact, communication and self-soothing. And these elements are extremely necessary for every human being, independent of his/her condition and personality. Jung helps me to understand the importance of human contact and communication for every personality when he says that we are isolated through our technical, rationally thinking civilization and through the loss of contact with nature. The original, pure acceptance of nature and its conditions served to integrate every human into society and into the whole cosmos. But we in the Western world are becoming 'dehumanized,' he says, through the increasing isolation from the natural laws.

> Thunder is no longer the voice of an angry god, nor is lightning his avenging missile. No river contains a spirit, no tree is the life principle of a man, no snake the embodiment of wisdom, no mountain cave the home of a great demon. No

> voices now speak from man to stones, plants, and animals, nor does he speak to them believing they can hear. His contact with nature has gone, and with it has gone the profound emotional energy that this symbolic connection supplied (Jung, 1964, p. 95).

Isolation is becoming a 'normal' problem in our present society. Many people suffer from it in the form of depression, neurosis, loneliness, and other psychological and physical handicaps. This sort of disintegration in the cosmos makes the distances between human beings and their environment seem irreconcilable. Every emotional contact, when not deeply connected to the original source of nature itself, can create problems.

Psychotherapist Janov describes the possible reconnection to emotional energy of suppressed feelings by expressing "primal screams." This type of therapy involves the client in reliving earliest memories by calling out to invisible parents for help and thus relieving the primal pains of childhood. Calling out like a child, screaming or yelling for parents to hear, help, comfort or just answer is very significant. If a child was not heard, helped, comforted or answered, primal pain builds up. Janov portrays these primal pains as feelings, which are essential for human life. If expression of feelings as a child is unwelcome or deprived–by not being allowed to cry when sad, for example–primal pain develops. "Feeling, then, is the antithesis of Pain," he says, and "the more pain one feels, the less pain one suffers" (1972, p. 101).

Through my work in psychiatric hospitals, I have met many disintegrated personalities. Isolation has manifested for some depressed or neurotic clients because of early 'imprisonment' of their archaic wishes and impulses of life. Often I have used my voice as a medium for primary contact from one human being to another and to reach the primal pains Janov describes. I have increased and later decreased tension to help clients re-experience vocally and bodily suppressed suffering through primal mourning, screaming, crying or calling out. From my personal natural source of emotional energy I have hoped that I could bridge their emotional block or prison. And when our voices resonated in the air between us, it also connected us with our environment.

THE ISOLATED VOICE – A CASE EXAMPLE

With one psychiatric client, a young intelligent woman in her thirties named Monique who suffered from a chronic borderline personality disorder, I had to use an unusual vocal approach. As every attempt to let Monique sing traditionally and participate in the music therapy group failed, her fear blocked her more and more. When Monique found it impossible to do simple vocal warm-ups or sing songs in a small group of traumatized woman, she became silent. Her usual voice was soft and fading out; she was blocked and frozen in her massive overweight body and fearful mind. I interpreted her frozen physical and emotional condition as a defence mechanism for her solitude. No other exercise, no talk, and no music could comfort her when she was in her normal daily fear. She insisted continuing the music sessions, telling me that she loved singing and music, unable to participate in anything else, but searching for help with her fear and panic attacks. Normally she exploded silently during her panic attacks when the fear became too strong, and often she destroyed objects. Sometimes even during treatment meetings, Monique would take any object and throw it on the floor–her signal to stop and to show that it was unbearable.

I had to create another workable form, a safer environment, taking Monique out of the group and starting individual sessions and asking her what she wanted to do. She offered me a method she recently had discovered: Tai-Chi breathing exercises. Empowering her, we began the session standing together with a warm-up breathing practice consisting of simultaneous rhythmic patterns of inhaling and exhaling. We gradually moved to making primal vocal sounds during the exhale, such as sighs. We incorporated synchronized body movement for support with swinging arms and stamping feet. Progressively we uttered natural sounds, which escaped our bodies organically. While I followed the intensive speed of our body movements, I encouraged deeper exhalations and louder wheezing and puffing. Communicating through our rhythmic breath and tone we represented forms of symbolic attachment and attunement, something that I cannot describe. Modulating between our bodily tensions and relaxation, Monique started painful screeching. Unexpectedly, she broke out into intense authentic screams, screaming with such a power as if she had to protect herself in front of a group of dangerous enemies. I instinctively screamed with her to fortify a 'wall of noise' as protection, matching her patterns and speed. We both screamed for at least 10 or 15 minutes, connected through such a vibrational understanding. The intensity of our screams bonded us together, supporting each other's instinctive, animalistic part of our personalities.

My colleagues came running to the room when they heard our voices to check if everything was okay. I was shocked and a bit ashamed because we sounded like two wild animals united in a shrieking sound. Giving nonverbal signs to my colleagues that we were okay, I continued without further explanation, careful not to break the cohesive emotional energy we had developed. Through our screaming, Monique became ready to get in contact with parts of her existential fear, maybe her shadow voice, the primal pains of her childhood. To touch this frightened terrain, she needed a simple form, a constructive framework in which to express her aggression. She did not panic or seem to be confused, but seriously focused herself onto this emotional discharge. Screaming together was an extraordinarily intimate experience and I cannot remember having done this before with anybody. Being able to share this created an illumination and empowerment. Whatever it was for Monique, it was the only helpful, relaxing and comforting form of emotional expression she permitted herself–at least for this moment.

Immediately following this tough, vital, vocal exercise, and after we relaxed while sitting down, I sang a soft improvisation to her as if she were a child: soothing, calming and comforting her. To create a safe place for her I sang without musical accompaniment about imaginary places in nature. During my improvisation I asked Monique to see herself sitting in the grass and enjoying being in the nature . . . imagine the flowers are growing . . . smell and fly with the fresh wind of the air . . . listen and sing with the birds. She calmed down and followed my directed imagery, a structure I used every time after her energetic vocal outbursts. I guided her, softly singing, through landscapes where she could find herself in a peaceful environment. I took time to support Monique's orientation into nature and places she needed to create for herself. After 5 or 10 minutes I guided her back into the situation of the music therapy room. The process of reorientation required care because of her fragile feelings of safety. Similar to a lullaby nurturing the mother-child relationship, I vocally comforted her. I felt that the vocal therapy form I developed at that moment did comfort her. But would it work again? Like discovering that we both spoke the same foreign language, our vocal sharing created a surprising intimacy that would take time to understand and integrate.

Instinctively we had created a ritual for the expression of existential fear as well as nurturing comfort. Monique told her psychotherapist, my colleague, about our 'ritual' as a form that helped her to express her emotions: being angry, being small and sorrowful like a child, and increasingly finding herself. Being able to share this experience with him opened a new space in her treatment. She included him as witness of her feelings about being small like a child, a fact that she always appreciated in sessions with me. The mother-child relationship I transferred during my sessions seemed closer to reality than I thought; and sharing anger together took on the nature of siblings, as well.

Monique had never screeched or screamed before, living a life with a non-expressive, isolated personality. Only when the tension got too high and she broke objects, did the little barbarians in her basement become active and suddenly destructive, as Wilber said. After I had acknowledged the intensity of our screams together, I realized that she benefited from this and we continued on a weekly basis. After weeks of regularly scheduled vocal outbursts she learned that she could structure her anger in a more contained form than breaking objects. The need to break disappeared and her fear diminished, giving me the impression that a small sense of safety had grown. Moving from the hospital to a protected, outpatient home enabling her to live by herself, was a significant step toward more independence. The beginning of liberation was seen through showing and sharing her childish, frightful, angry girl–the shadow side of her grown-up personality.

Monique was the first client I was consciously aware of who had awakened the little barbarians in myself in the course of doing therapy. I discovered that our voices together had a strong impact on me, too. Being comfortable with my own voice through years of voicework training, I now found myself needing to use it for the extremes of rough and shrill roaring in every session. Monique needed the initial outburst to contact her Self and to break through the walls of her isolation. Mirroring her archaic wishes and impulses of life the energy moved through her voice out into the world.

Chapter III

In this chapter I focus on the deepest, most spontaneous form of vocal human expression for pain, anger, grief or happiness in the form of *Acoustic Symbols.* As 'eternal truth' (according to Jung), symbols deserve correct understanding, preservation and integration. Acoustic symbols that are deeply understood carry the vocal potential of comfort, as with a lullaby that integrates an improvised melody around a baby's cry. *Maternal Voices* explores the research of Jayne M. Standley and others around vocal sounds beneficial for growth and development in prematurely born babies. In *Primitive Voices*, I explore Annette Cramer's preverbal musical babbling sounds combined with simple musical elements that portray primitive melodies as cure in a cultural perspective. The technique of using the human voice for medical assessment and treatment is highlighted through Joanne Loewy's tonal and language development work to engender wisdom and understanding of those sounds. In *The Excited Voice* I dialogue with a nonverbal autistic boy by breaking into the aloneness of his cries, excited babbles, or anxious screams in a special education setting.

ACOUSTIC SYMBOLS

The authentic human behavior of making natural sounds can be found everywhere in life today but as I said before, often we limit, suppress or don't hear it. People express joy and pain, making bright and dark sounds, and through this they make a connection with their environment. Through these sounds they are creating acoustic symbols for pain, anger, grief or happiness–the deepest, most spontaneous form of emotional expression. This expression is the indication of their feeling, spirit and character at the moment. It is the intonation of their most personal reaction, the quality and power of their emotion, clearly audible through the voice. The act of expressing and not limiting or suppressing these human sounds presents them as meaningful symbols. These symbols develop over time a complexity of associated meanings and inherent values. Wolfsohn experienced many of these authentic sounds in the First World War and understood them as meaningful symbols. And like him, I am convinced that everybody is able to understand these human acoustic symbols naturally and interact with them as people have through the centuries.

Jung wrote about the importance of symbols in a traditional visual way, and about the preservation and integration of them in society. He described symbols as vehicles for expressing eternal truths that have been transformed by long processes of emotional, social and cultural development. Conscious or not, these symbols have become collective truths that are accepted by societies.

Acoustic symbols, like Jung's archetypal symbols, are also universally accepted truths. Some acoustic symbols can evoke a deep emotional response in individuals and we have to be alert to recognize and understand them. If just as some visual symbols their 'eternal truths' are neglected by civilized societies, then there is the danger that their specific energy might disappear. Once we have lost them to the unconscious, there will be unaccountable consequences. Jung is concerned about the strong impact of rationalization and the loss of moral and spiritual traditions, the isolation of human beings, and their distance from nature. And he thinks that symbols and their recognition and understanding are able to exert beneficial influences on the unconscious.

In this discussion of acoustic symbols, I would like to adopt Jung's idea about the importance of preserving and integrating symbols. The loss of connection and integration with nature makes us strangers also to our own authentic sounds whether expressing themselves as universal acoustic symbols or in uniquely personal ways. The sounds of acoustic symbols in the world seem to be similar everywhere: a painful groan in Africa sounds the same as in Europe; a happy cheer is the same for people in Asia and America and Africa; the words may be different but the intonation is the same. There will be different codes for expressions, languages and enormous cultural distinctions between people of different continents, but these pure acoustic symbols are not unique; instead they express the 'eternal truths.' They are a trans-cultural as well as a paralinguistic vocabulary universal in human existence. Through these paralinguistic expressions we learn how uniform the original sounds really are and we can see them as archetypes of human expression.

Newham describes them as acoustic symbols, and he inspired me to think more about them as symbols for all human beings:

> These acoustic symbols of 'vital consciousness,' which, we may speculate, were once expressed through the spontaneous vocal sounds of early peoples and later formed the core of primitive song, compare to the preverbal musical babblings of the infant, as though each new born child in a matter of months traces the development of human beings played out over thousands of years (Newham, 1989, p. 156).

If we follow acoustic symbols as empirical treasures of human existence, the impact of those babblings and cries appear to be tremendous. In simple historical perspective we could believe that acoustic symbols are witnesses of forms of human development. As I explained in the previous chapter about the importance of primal screams, the emotional and physical impact of being allowed to make sounds during childhood is tremendous. The creation of 'primal pains' (as Janov called them) starts when those sounds are suppressed, somewhere forcing and delaying human development.

MATERNAL VOICES

If I follow this comparison between acoustic symbols and the sounds babies make, I conceive that the acoustic symbol of an adult cry of pain and the babbling of an infant are both healthy behaviors and as such are examples of authentic individual, paralinguistic expression. I, as a human being, can understand the sound of a baby even without being a parent. More difficult for me is to understand when the baby has problems. But for the baby's mother or father understanding the meaning of various cries comes more naturally. An intense bond between baby and parent makes the communication easy. This communication is so intense because of their close connection; mother and baby originally shared the same body and the baby is identified with the mother, with her sound, smell, movement and touch. The father's presence and voice are likewise valuable for creating contact. Through their bodies and the well-known sounds of their voices, parent and baby experience intimate sensations and assimilate them as vital consciousness. A symbiotic relationship builds up if that relationship is an exchange of intensive intimate information between two humans.

In very early research studies from the thirteenth century, experiments were conducted to discover the influence of the contact between mothers and their babies. In a study under Emperor Friedrich II in Europe (Cramer), mothers were taken away from their newborn babies and replaced with deaf, nonverbal nannies. These nannies were told to cover their faces and to avoid any kind of social or emotional contact, sounds and gestures with the babies. The babies only received routine feeding and necessary changing activities. Babies receiving this treatment died after a short time. This human research example would not be possible to repeat today but it demonstrates the intense, vital relationship between mothers and babies. Harlow's well-known study about monkeys and the replacement of their feeding mothers with substitutes, showed similar results. Harlow's experiments might be questionable today, too, but we can learn from both the importance of physical and vocal contact for early bonding[8].

---

8. Harlow separated a baby monkey from its mother and raised it in a cage with two substitute "mothers." There was a wire "mother" with a bottle for the infant, and a cloth one without a bottle. Tellingly, as soon as the infants finished nursing they abandoned the wire monkey and clutched the

Through the work of music therapists in Neonatal Intensive Care Units (NICU), we have learned that premature babies may after birth benefit from the sound of their mother's voice and the rhythm of womb-sounds to which the fetus has become accustomed (Collins & Kuck, 1991). In different research studies around the world, premature babies were treated with singing by a female voice to improve oxygen saturation and stimulate the sucking reflex. Jayne M. Standley, for example, emphasized at the Ninth World Congress for Music Therapy in 1999 the role of music in pacification/stimulation of premature infants with low birth weights, and how the singing female voice typically stimulated the reflexes of premature babies around the age of 34 weeks. As Standley detailed in her book (2003), through exposures to soft singing, the researchers in NICU tried to bring the babies from a hyper-position–resulting from too early separation from mother's body–to a homeostasis and to help decrease their stress level. First the non-nutritive sucking reflex was activated and then babies learned how to suck in general. So they were stimulated to be active and later even gained weight and could go home earlier.

Standley says that an infant's preferred order of auditory stimulus is: 1) the mother's voice; 2) if the mother is not available, then another female voice; and 3) finally, music. Other research shows that babies recognize the mother's voice when exposed to other female voices. Female voices seem to have a unique quality of a warm, high, emotional sound, covering the baby like a blanket. Male voices–such as the father's or the sound of siblings–can develop into a familiar and comforting sound environment in which the baby can re-connect to sounds it heard as a fetus. But the mother's voice is very significant for the baby to recognize and bond with. In the NICU, reading, talking or singing lullabies during visits, or playing recordings of the mother's voice, are helpful ways to support bonding for the baby. Research also shows that listening to lullabies promotes language development in infants.

Nöcker-Ribaupierre (2003) collected international music therapy approaches in the Neonatal Intensive Care Unit (NICU) and published an amazing treasure of research. Various beneficial sound stimulations are presented, but the significant role of the mother's voice in connection with early intervention as well as long-term effects on development is emphasized. Pain management, speech development, increased language understanding and intensive bonding are only some of the benefits she describes.

In a pilot study Nöcker-Ribaupierre demonstrated the long-term effect of vocal sound on prematurely born babies. Exposed to 30 minutes of recordings

---

cloth one. Even though the experiment demonstrated the primacy of nurturing to sustenance, the cloth mother was not an adequate replacement: the isolated monkeys grew up with severe emotional and behavioral problems, says Carlson, associate professor of neuroscience and psychology at Harvard Medical School (1999, http://whyfiles.org/087mother/4.html and http://users.rcn.com/napier.interport/cwm/experim.html).

of their mothers' voices five times a day in the incubator, babies in an experimental group relaxed and increased their oxygen saturation. Nöcker-Ribaupierre compared this group with a control group, which did not receive any specific forms of stimulation. The long-term effect was measured after 5 and 20 months, and after 4.8 and 6.3 years. After 5 months the experimental group showed significant progress in verbal and motor development. After 20 months and 4.8 years this difference was still recognized but not significant. At the age of 6.3 years the HSET[9] speech test showed significant advances in understanding speech and language in the experimental group. These studies also demonstrated improvements in the mother-child relationship as evidenced by and increase of 50% vs. 12.5% more breastfeeding and psychic stability by both mother and baby.

Another unconscious practice of mothers is also fascinating: holding their babies on the left side of their body while breast-feeding them reinforces the comforting effect of the heartbeat heard for nine months in the womb. Early attachment and attunement through sound and rhythm show the intense contact babies establish with their environment. The process of emotional and physical bonding has its roots in those early connections where human contact and interaction start. In various research studies about songs for children, the structure of a lullaby, for example, was found to be the same in nearly every culture: a slow rhythm and a simple repetitive pattern for the melody, small intervals, with few harmonic changes in the course of the song.

> It may have its origin in onomatopoeia[[10]] because it is easy to imagine a parent improvising a melody for a distressed child, or a sleepy one, uttering no more words than 'la-la-la' [. . .] Lullabies may be particularly effective, because, in general, they combine the benefits of the female voice in a simple orchestrated format (Schwartz & Ritchie, 1999, p. 18).

Independent of the language, climate or other influences, the lullaby, often sung by female voices with a simple melody and repetitive rhythm, had a soothing, relaxing effect and has been used in both early and contemporary cultures. In modern times, the nurturing male voice has become more common as fathers have increasingly taken on the role of supportive caregiver. These spontaneous vocal sounds show an aspect of the development of human beings–female and male–as natural caregivers through the form of a primitive song.

9. HSET Heidelberger Sprachentwiclungstest = Heidelberger speech development test
10. Onomatopoeia: formation of a word by imitation of a sound made by or associated with its referent (Stein, 1966, *The Random Dictionary*).

PRIMITIVE VOICES

Primitive forms of comfort and cure for babies, infants, and adults are very similar from one culture to the next. The repetitive, simple form of singing, as in the lullaby, is significant for diverse cultures. Newham and Cramer (1998) quote a variety of music history sources to define and describe the aspect of repetition in primitive music for different ethnic groups. Both talk about a connection between the 'babble songs' of infants and primitive music, and point out the extremely repetitive patterns of both. It is possible that this does not apply to all cultures, but many researchers have explored the appearance of very simple melodies and rhythms that are repeated successively in many forms of primitive music.

A 'primitive melody' is no more than a continually repeated and varied motif. Additionally, the emotionality and timbre of the vocal style relates more to the meaning than the compositional structure of the melody. In many comparable studies the similarity was shown between the structure of the babble sound of an infant and original, primitive music. Cramer used an example of Klusen in her book about the voice to show, through the simplicity of a melody, how the two parallel each other–the babble sound of infant and primitive music–to create a relaxing effect. She believes that when the melody has a strong relaxing impact, it should be made of as few tones as possible. This minimal melody, called a 'centric melody,' was found all over the world, and everywhere structured in the same way: centered around one tone as melodic germ cell. The 'centric melody' was used in ancient songs with a strong repetitive character in which the singer stabilized his intonation through bodily movement: stamping, bending or dancing to deepen the body connection. The repetition and movement were also needed to intensify the mental and physical experience so as to finally induce trance states.

On the next page are several examples of simple melodic lines of original primitive music and the preverbal musical babbling sound or scream structure of infants (Cramer, p. 214). In each of these melodies are acoustic symbols collected and musically annotated, and we can learn to recognize them through understanding their context. I believe that simple vocal melodies of primitive music and vocal expressions of infants are extremely important human sounds. The property of repetition in both helps us to understand their natural pacifying effect. It calls for understanding the incredibly meaningful messages of this transcultural phenomenon within the environment and the society.

Healing melody of the Taulipang, America

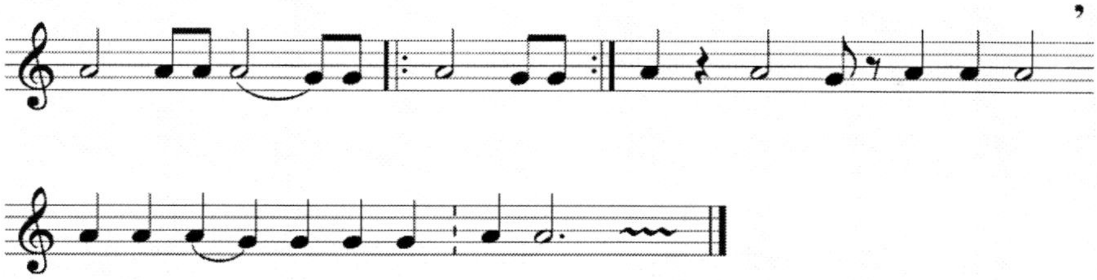

Healing-blessing-formula, Germany

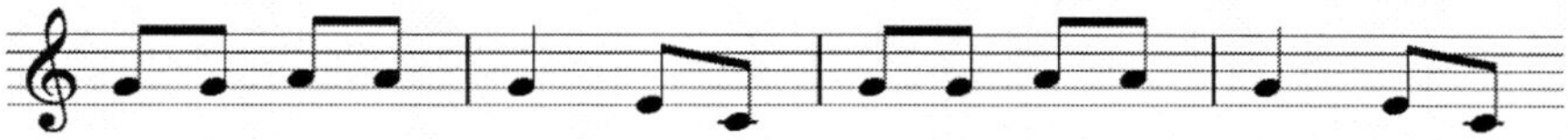

Shamanistic song in healing ritual

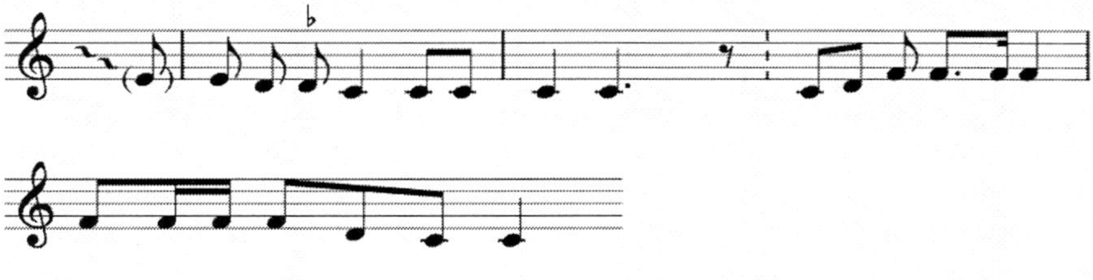

Transposed babble or domesticated scream structure of an infant

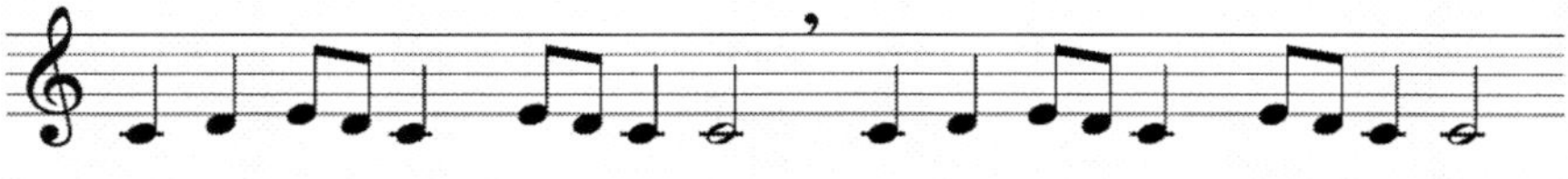

What we have learned about the lullaby as a mother's reaction to the infant's babble we can intensify and apply to other sounds such as the cry or the scream. Joanne V. Loewy (1995, 2004) studied the development of language

and the preverbal sounds of children and is a pioneer in this field. She brings awareness into these ignored communicative qualities of infant cries: it is a "remarkably efficient signal, which indicates that the baby is hungry, cold, lonely or in distress," quoting Oswald. In the same article she describes offered support to enhance: crying to comfort, babble to lull, and word or speech development through music therapy, encouraging vocal mirroring of infant sounds:

> In inflected vocal play, no words involved. Communicative vocalizations are reinforced through the inherently musical elements of the cry. Music therapists often sing in a child's tonality, mirroring the baby's sound that in turn provide refuge in resolving cries of distress (2004, Integrating Music, Language and the Voice in Music Therapy).

Loewy supports research of Briggs (1991) that brings to light–through studies done by Fridman and Oswald about vocal/tonal development–more information about the recorded voices of infants. Fridman pointed out that the "newborn cry is made up of five to twelve contiguous sounds that are repeated. By 4 months, infants' voices are firmer and their range extends an octave more than at birth." Oswald "described the neonatal cry as a regular sequence of tones in a rising and falling pattern with the maximum loudness around 60 decibels." Furthermore he "observed that pain or distress increase the duration and loudness and elevate the pitch of the cry" (Briggs, p. 4-5).

Loewy analysed the child's voice to indicate normal and abnormal development, diagnosis, and other problems the child may be experiencing. Loewy refers to other research in which the child's cry was analysed. A weak whine could show a closeness of Tay Sach's[11] symptoms, or a high, sharp, staccato crying could possibly give an idea about brain defects or severe brain damage or meningitis. Those sounds might become increasingly important for future development of diagnosis and treatment. And the treasures of the countless recordings from Nordoff-Robbins Center for Music Therapy[12] show the significance of vocal sounds such as crying, screaming, or sing-crying as forms of primitive expression. Robbins used the term 'primal aria' for it because he heard in their singing an authentically pure and dramatically strong expression of an emotional need to which he musically responded.

11.Tay-Sachs disease, a rare, fatal disease occurring chiefly in infants and children, is characterized by a red spot on the retina, gradual blindness, and loss of weight, and believed to be of genetic origin (Stein, 1966, *The Random Dictionary*).
12. Nordoff-Robbins Center for Music Therapy worldwide; UK, USA, Australia, Germany, Japan. Search for case 'Edward.'

During a curious study about the human scream in the year 2000, I measured the screaming voices of healthy female and male adults in a relaxed but concentrated situation. I found out that these screams were repetitive, used many sliding tones as well as microtones, and their ranges extended through intensity of the sound. After the screamers repeated their individual patterns of screaming several times, they filtered out the cognitive intention, moved into the emotion of their bodies, and used the voice-as-being. Their screams then sounded like screams of babies. Is it possible through screaming to really reconnect oneself to the primary energy of a baby, to this emotional energy (see *Shadowed Voices*, Janov)? And is it possible to treat adult screams the same as baby ones? All of those research studies look at the cry or scream in a musical context, which is what the mother's lullaby and a shaman's song are contributing intuitively to comfort human beings.

In different research studies it was found that the structure of babies' nonverbal expressions is the same in every culture because of the presumably identical babble sounds infants create. Independent of the culture and language, babies generate the same language exercises to train all of the articulation zones for development of vowels and consonants. Every baby starts with 'a,' 'aba' or 'papapa' and 'mamama' sounds, articulated through the lips which are connected to the suck reflex. Babies have a universal language, Chomsky said, made up of structures which are inherent in their genes (Cramer). Parents in every culture and language are able to understand these archetypical expressions independent of their own background and can translate them into their language or dialects.

Could it be that people in every culture intuitively adapted the simple structure of a lullaby to the infant's own repertoire of sound? Probably there is a unique interchange of emotions, information, and sound, with also an archetypical understanding of their environment. This interchange is intensely assuring, rooted in the tradition of human beings existing in every culture, language and oral, musical tradition–not only between babies and their environment. I maintain that this phenomenon exists also between grown-ups and their cultural environment, and this is what I want to explore in the following chapters about forms of primitive singing.

Through these vibrant vocalizations people are interacting with each other, adapting and integrating their acoustic symbols into a vital consciousness within society. We can benefit from learning more about primitive cultures and their need for exchange of those individual and social expressions. Would this authentic vocal interaction and the unique behavior of different cultures show us the real potential of the human voice? Listening carefully to these original sounds of vocal interaction and music personally helps me to better understand human beings, to realize how we have limited ourselves in our highly civilized world, and also to appreciate the potential we still carry with us. We did not lose it but we do not use it! Our new challenge could be threefold: to learn that this type of communication with nature, with ourselves and each other is possible through the sound of our voices; to learn more about ourselves through forms of trance, attachment and security, and discovering subpersonalities; and to re-connect with our spiritual, personal, and social environments.

Kate Richards Geller (1997) wrote about the importance of singing, toning and chanting in music therapy for pain management with children. For her, singing with a child's cry engenders a give-and-take exchange, a musical internal and external mirror of human pain. In the same book, Rothenberg described the unity when two voices come together: "when one naked human howl meets another, the walls are gone" (Rothenberg in Richards Geller, p. 69). I believe here is the entrée to a real therapeutic relationship. Any age child with limited language skills can demonstrate that there are multifunctional sounds with important meanings, just as I explained earlier about the babies.

So often I have experienced the established unity of two voices in my work. I am still astonished about it. Once in a group session with 6-year-olds, I stopped the song I was singing and interacted with one child who had suddenly broken out in a cry. I vocally matched the pattern of the cry rhythmically and tonally, using no words and moving into a simple (centric) melody. The child's cry became more structured, first intensive in tone and later softer in volume. Singing that way made me feel relaxed and comfortable and better able to soothe the child. This must be similar to what mothers experience while vocally calming their child. The other children in the group were astonished and silent; every child was listening intently while I continued singing to the child who, bit by bit, became tranquil. It seemed to me that the other children were affected too–calmed and relaxed because the cry was held through my voice instead of stopped while disturbing the group.

Breaking musically into the aloneness of a cry, sigh, babble or anxious breath can be so influential and effective that we need to be more attentive to it. Our voices carry the simplicity of a powerful tool, a tool for navigation and for treatment.

THE EXCITED VOICE – A CASE EXAMPLE

David–a small, shy, very sensitive, autistic, nonverbal 9-year-old boy I worked with for two years in the School for Children with Special Needs–was well known for being extremely aggressive. He hid his face when in contact with others, put his arm around his head, covered his face, and avoided looking at and being seen by others. He could suddenly, without provocation, attack somebody in the room, hitting or slamming into children and adults, pulling hair or clothes and throwing furniture. He had limited verbal skills; he only used long and loud screams during his attacks, babbled and hummed when relaxed and uttered high vocal sounds to express excitement and pleasure. I worked with him individually each week to address his extreme, aggressive behaviour.

David's interesting vocal expressions and his love for music were beneficial for making contact during music therapy. He sat on a chair or stood in a corner, touching the floor with his hands or hiding his face, looking briefly under his covered arm in my direction while he was listening to the music I played. He rarely touched an instrument or interacted musically with me. If I got up from my place at the keyboard and came closer to him, he would push me back with his hands. He did not push or hit me aggressively, but he made clear that I should not be close to him. Whenever he touched an instrument he would make excited vocal sounds. I accepted his anxiety and need for distance, gave him space and time to meet me musically when he was ready.

One of the most significant moments of contact between David and me occurred after 5 months of work. He threw the mallets of the xylophone in my direction and then softly pushed me in the same direction. I did not see this as an aggressive attack but as an attempt to make contact with me in a very safe way. I picked the mallets up, made a vocal sound similar to him and gave the mallets back. He smiled and seemed to like my reaction. He did it again and we got into a playful game that he repeated over and over. He enjoyed seeing me picking up the mallets, making exciting vocal sounds and giving them back. This became a ritual for us for the next months and David demanded that I followed his game, satisfying his obsessive autistic behaviour. For a while I continued this ritual, and later I tried to introduce small changes or adaptations.

Generally I tried to match his sounds with my own voice, singing around his tones, singing his name or simple ostinato patterns and improvising melodies. The acoustic symbols of his sound were mirrored, contained, pacified or provoked. I believe that our vocal contact must have made him feel heard, comforted or stimulated, in the sense of "when one naked human howl meets another, the walls are gone." I honestly felt that I communicated with him, echoing his sounds or varying around his patterns, using his vocalizations and expressions as entrance for contact. The practice of exchanging our acoustic symbols made me believe that we performed the universal form of expression. Transforming his authentic sounds into a musical context, creating simple melodic patterns with repetition, became our vocal dialogue.

The following musical passage is a part of our good-bye song where David vocally dialogued with me, imitated and completed my musical phrases. Imagining this boy as autistic and extremely violent, unable to express verbally any of his needs and feelings, our musical conversation was a bridge into this limitation. His excited voice was humming, murmuring or just singing around my sounds. He communicated in and around my pitch, created melodic motifs and rhythmical phrases like a second voice, and he offered his own variations. While he vocally expressed his unique personality and communicated with me, his pleasure and enthusiasm in being heard and mirrored resonated with us. The "music child" in him awoke, as Nordoff/Robbins called the unknown musicality that every child carries. I can only imagine that sharing such emotional contact made a profound impact on him.

After 6 month's of work David interacted with me, vocalized, moved my hands on the keyboard and played it himself. I understood his gestures as a sign that I should continue playing. He rocked in the rhythm that we were playing on keyboard and he vocally expressed being excited about it or he imitated my sounds. I believe we had built up a level of understanding which created safety, allowing him to become more comfortable and trusting of me.

Once he became angry and violent, threw the cymbal on the ground, started running around room, pulling paper from the walls and tried to attack me. I remained still and quietly spoke to him, saying, "It is ok to be confused about the noise from outside." I tried to hold his hands but he bit me and I let go but did not punish him. While I was putting each instrument away I kept talking with a quiet, low voice to him. I reassured him that he would be okay and he could calm down. Lastly I sang relaxing sounds, long 'ahhh's' accompanied by minor keys on the keyboard, using a simple melody. He calmed down and moved into his protected posture, possibly expecting more danger and punishment as was usual in the classroom.

Minutes later he was in fear and panic and lost control again and screaming, threw the keyboard from the stand aggressively, making a crashing sound. This time I clearly said "NO" louder to stop more violence, but I did not scream at him. Here was my audible boundary and I set my limit. I took time to relax myself while David was reacting to what happened around him. He did not attack the instruments and me again and I waited for his relaxation. Some minutes later I went with him to the keyboard to show him that he had to pick it up. He seemed to understand me and together we pulled the keyboard back on the stand and we cleaned up the room (nothing was broken!). Both of us were quiet and we left the room in silence; understanding each other on a primal level needed no words. His improvement in our nonverbal conversation was tremendous; he followed my hands guiding him into the classroom without any interruption. It seemed that the unique interchange of emotions, information, and sound had created an archetypical understanding of each other and of our environment.In the sessions following this violent incident, David showed more tenderness with me than he ever did before. He came into the room smiling, walked straight to keyboard and sat on my lap, rocked back and forth loudly vocalizing while I was singing and playing to him. He gave me big hugs and did

Goodbye

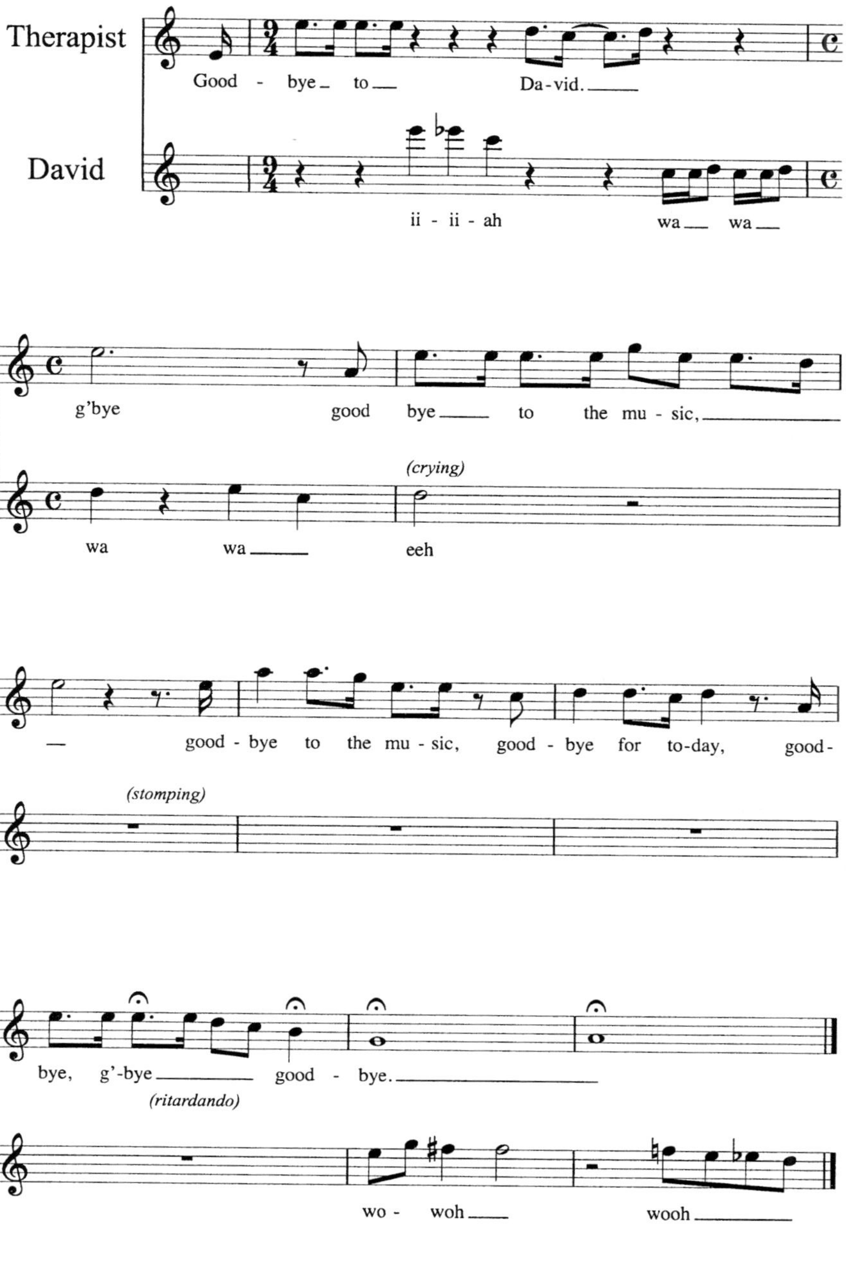
Therapist
Good - bye to Da-vid.
David
ii - ii - ah wa wa
g'bye good bye to the mu - sic,
(crying)
wa wa eeh
good - bye to the mu - sic, good - bye for to-day, good-
(stomping)
bye, g'-bye good - bye.
(ritardando)
wo - woh wooh

Goodbye

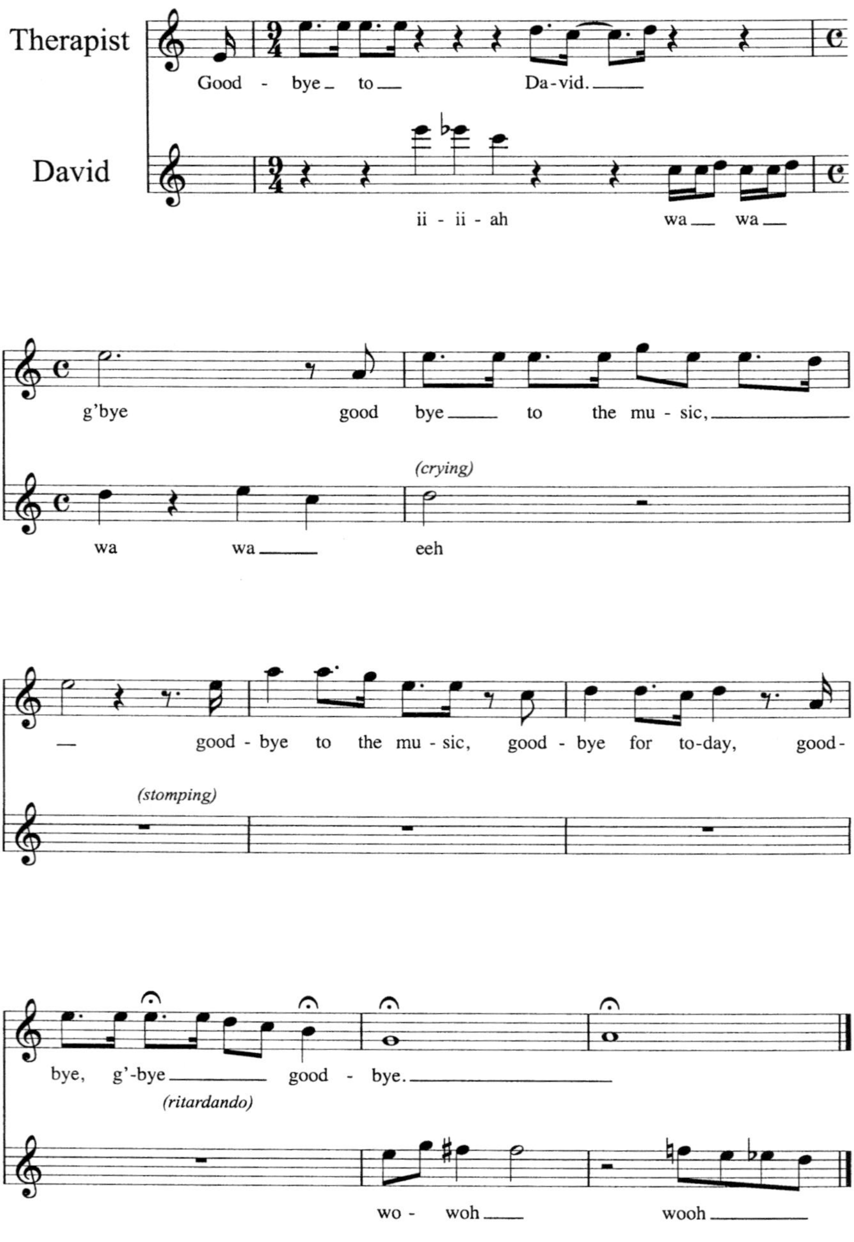
Therapist
David
Good - bye to Da-vid.
ii - ii - ah wa wa
g'bye good bye to the mu - sic,
(crying)
wa wa eeh
good - bye to the mu - sic, good - bye for to-day, good-
(stomping)
bye, g'-bye good - bye.
(ritardando)
wo - woh wooh

not want to leave the area around the keyboard where I was sitting. When he hung his whole body over the edge of the chair or over my lap, I touched his back, softly singing about him in a lullaby form. It seemed like he needed more emotional contact, similar to an infant discovering affection. Unexpectedly he would jump up, run away and come back with his excited vocal sounds, hugging me. Autistic children have to go through those emotional stages step by step as all children do. Even as a 9-year-old his emotional development seemed to start with me from the baby stage and move gradually to higher levels as I explained also in the case in Chapter I concerning the developmental stages of children.

Again, after a while he needed to turn away briefly and come back with open arms or put his lips on my cheek as if kissing. During these excited active moments he looked at me, laughed or smiled and made his high vocal sounds which I matched vocally through improvisations in the same key.David was experiencing bonding through our treasured vocal interventions and musical contact as well as discovering his own need for personal space. In one session he was sitting on my lap at the keyboard as we were finishing up an active musical collaboration. While I was still playing and singing a song he put both of his arms around my neck, pulled me gently close to his head and held my head there for a long while. Touched by his intimate attempt, I switched the text of the song I was singing from "there is a little wheel in my heart" to "there is a little boy in my heart." As if he understood the meaning of the words he pulled my head closer to him, keeping intimate contact with me. This need for making a profound emotional connection seemed new for him and I changed my singing to lullaby sounds of rocking a baby, using no words, only open vocal sounds. To give him more time for discovery and myself space to process this surprising reaction, I continued singing that way. He held himself physically close to me, giving me the impression that he had found what he was searching for. It is difficult for autistic children to build up any emotional attachment, and this seemed an important breakthrough for him.

Our work benefited from his intensive emotional and musical contact. His high excited sounds became the significant symbol of our contact. But also our silent or intuitive understanding of each other showed similarity to the primal mother-child connection. I truly believe that his level of understanding his environment had been improved. Often he came close to me and hugged me, and regularly he accepted my roles, restrictions and changes without being angry. Discovery of new instruments with different fine motor requirements and more engagement with me became a new focus. During our two years together I saw his inflexible behaviour change and I experienced no aggressive attacks. The classroom teacher recognized a huge decrease of his aggression from one or two tantrums a day the previous year to one a week. In school David was getting recognized for his new emotional and social skills and he was gradually able to tolerate and contact others more easily. Years after our therapy I met David again. His teacher told me that his tantrums had entirely disappeared, and he was unable to imagine that this boy had ever had aggressive outbursts.

His pleasure in making natural sounds, expressing joy and being silent after moments of panic, making bright and dark sounds, and through this making a connection with his environment, was as essential for David as it is for other human beings. Through these sounds children and adults around the world create their acoustic symbols for pain, anger, grief or happiness, symbols that are recognizable in every culture of human existence.

Chapter IV

In an analysis of the origin of language as a form of human expression with its cultural differences, this chapter investigates intercultural forms of vocal communication and understanding. In *Cultural Voices* I describe Paul Moses's vocal differentiations across cultures and other characteristic female/male examples from Western and Middle Eastern origin. *Linguistic Voices* puts vocal sounds under the microscope of developed dialects and languages and looks at vocal creativity around the world. As humans migrate and travel, languages split, proliferate and transform. In *My Multicultural Voice* I describe my own personal vocal, musical, political, spiritual, and cultural transformation as a result of shifting languages, cultures and music. *The Foreign Voice* portrays my visit to Turkey, where I vocally comforted a handicapped girl in a language I didn't understand.

CULTURAL VOICES

Where does the voice come from? Everybody is born with a voice as a natural, biological instrument, which is becoming a cultural phenomenon through its adaptations. The voice becomes the most personal symbol of a human organism, reflecting its culture and finally human development at large. The voice develops and changes from a childish voice to an adult voice, a young voice to an old voice, and certainly from a natural voice to a more forced one, maybe a native-speaking to a foreign-speaking voice. These cultural influences seem to determine the sound of the voice, but not the deepest, most spontaneous form of its emotional expression.

Moses (1954) wrote about different vocal sounds and ranges across cultures. He noticed that all civilized people in the world today have narrowed their vocal range for speaking, but within various cultures considerable differences have developed. He observed among Oriental people (possibly meaning the Middle East and parts of Asia), that singing and speaking are distinctly separate functions; singing is high, speaking is low. He discovered that there also seem to be some geographical distinctions. Using the Equator as the line between north and south, there seems to be higher male and lower female voices in the south. Some languages offer greater vocal freedom than others; Italian, for example, uses wider ranges in daily dialogue than Scottish. Not only do greater ranges exist between languages but also there are enormous variations within the dialects of any single language.

Observing Oriental singing and speaking voices, the total expression of the human creature is audible. Their voices may be utilized differently, with different range and tonal qualities, depending on the individual expressions of the person at the moment. The differences in pitch and idiom between the high singing and low speaking voice are significant in Oriental people. Through my own travels in the Middle East I have discovered some more unusual aspects. I felt that the women in the big cities of Turkey, for example, speak with higher voices than those in Northern Europe; more significantly, they speak differently from women in villages of the same country. Since they left their villages and live in the big cities, they possibly need more support for their personal survival because of the loss of some of their original feminine roles, which could be reflected through their voices. I imagine that the reason for this could be a sign of their new or assimilated dependency on whatever is needed to survive in a big city: jobs, men, and different clothes. Wearing high heel shoes, for example, might have a big impact on the way women walk and feel carrying their bodies. Leaving flat shoes, with contact to the ground through work in fields (a grounding aspect), the feeling of being 'lifted' up to high shoes could have 'lifted' their voices too and 'heightened' their sound. The need of supporting men to hold onto while walking on high heels, adjusting to dress codes or a job requiring 'being on top of the work' could influence their feeling about being female. The reality of losing contact with the ground could of itself serve to manipulate their vocal sounds.

Separated from their environment and natural activities such as farming, far from their surroundings and historical sceneries with rich ceremonies, these women could become dependent. Could it be that the lifestyle differences in cities forced them to adopt a new identity? Outside of cities, women are around the house in more traditional roles, are more connected with nature, and they have lower voices. Could it be an acoustic sign of change of personal and social identification that is audible in the voice and its civilization?

In Turkish and Middle Eastern music there exists another interesting phenomenon: low 'macho' speaking voices allow typically high-pitched male singing voices to express feminine sensitivity and subtlety. Only in singing is a high male voice accepted by the cultural roles of this society. Young men can walk hand in hand through the streets of Istanbul to show a kind of habitual 'brotherly friendship.' But if a young man openly shows his gay gender through a higher, softer speaking voice, feminine gestures or clothing, unless he is an artist, the society isolates him. Only for singers is it acceptable to exhibit their sensibility or femininity through their art. This society is now changing in the big cities, too, and the existence of homosexuality is being recognized and gradually accepted as it has been in Western cultures. This process could be an opportunity for a vigorous use of an expanded authentic voice, a natural expression for human capacities and gender-extending abilities. Humans are exceptionally adaptive to their environment and reflective of their inner potential, and this could be an extraordinary example.

The identification, imitation, archetypes, and mannerisms of the singing and speaking voice clearly show patterns of cultural preference. For example, to be kind means not to raise the voice in a civilized culture. A cultivated British accent is a perfect example of this kindness and of the restriction of any 'full-bodied,' untamed vocal sounds. Yet, a male voice from the Mediterranean area with a strong, gravely, masculine, 'macho' sound is intended to send power out, attracting males and females, and is accepted in this role.

Low male voices in Western society are the prototype of objective stability with monotone, minimal swaying or variations in their voices. The fear of losing their authentic low voices is recognizable in many jokes and anecdotes about the destiny and life stories of castrati singers, who lost their sexual and patriarchal potency. Or is this instead the cultural expression of homophobia?Female voices in industrialized societies try to follow this masculine preference. Women have conformed their sounds through the last decades to affect a lower register. This change may have happened because of the assumption that they will be better accepted in this male-dominated society if they do not sound so 'feminine.' In movies, radio, TV as well as in many professional settings the preference for low female voices is apparent. While traditionally the typical maternal voice is negatively identified with babbling sounds, noises, crying and high tones, the motherly caretaking voice is held in a positive light. Herein appears the aspect of the voice as a 'blanket' of comforting warm and high sounds with the identification of infantile scenes (see *Maternal Voices*). For professional settings, such as radio, TV and film this aspect of the female voice has limited use. Females have to adapt the sound of their voices constantly, changing from motherly sounds to serious professional sounds or even to sexually seducing sounds. The wish to be taken seriously in business with a seductive lower female voice has also a physical component. It resonates more strongly in the body and the masculine quality of the sound extends the gender identification.

These limitations or extensions of the voice are echoed through cultural dependence. It is conceivable also that temperature and climate have influences on the quality of the voice: the voice in a body in warmer countries would be more relaxed, expressive, melodic round; in colder ones perhaps more hard, less expressive and linear. I consider that in landscapes with mountains, the sound of the voice might have more ups and downs in the melody of the language than in flatlands. Listening to foreign languages sounds like listening to outlandish music; following its melodic and rhythmic lines seems like travelling over mountains and valleys.

Whenever we travel we can listen to the language we cannot understand, listen to the landscapes. Do those sounds fit with what we see, smell and experience? Consider the Australian aboriginals, who describe their landscapes through complex songs, singing with different pitches, reciting about their environment, mountain, desert and valleys. Through specific song-lines, vocal arpeggios tell about a peak, falling into monotone when the landscape is stretching widely. Precisely describing details of the landscape vocally, those songs where used as a map, a help for survival, giving direction in the endless landscape of Australia (see Appendix B).

LINGUISTIC VOICES

Languages have always been transformed and modified through the circumstances of the environment. All populations created their own languages through alteration and amendment. 100,000 years ago the first communicative language appeared in Eastern Africa. As humans travelled, languages split and proliferated. Today there are now around 5,000 languages, with a variety of 15 language families spread over all continents with countless treasures of sounds, all made originally by voices. The most widely represented family is the Indo-European, which includes the Germanic (English, German, Dutch), the Romance (Italian, French, Spanish), the Celtic (Welsh, Scots, Irish), the Slavic (Russian, Polish, Slovenian), and the Indo-Iranian (Persian, Hindi, Kurdish). This is an incomplete list but it gives an idea of some audible connections and differences between America, Europe and Asia.

A language is a living experience because humans need it to communicate with each other in all stages of life. Therefore no communities, so far, have been found without some form of a language. The same is true for music. Every language has its own complexity, and linguists discern that there are no 'simple' languages. Their complexity can differ from others but all have their own expressive power, vocabulary, sounds, symbols and special use, created by the voices of human beings.

One interesting aspect for the specific creativity of human beings is the purposeful production of words, vocal and musical sounds, and grammar. For example, bridging huge distances, people found the practical solution of 'Jodeln,' yodel a form of singing language and communication in mountainous areas, combining high and low sounds of the voice through switches in between the vocal registers. While well known in the Alps of Europe, it is found also in two different continents without any cultural connections: Siberia in Asia and in mountainous Africa[13].

A different way mountains can determine language qualities is with the languages of the Basques in the Pyrenees, between Spain and France. The Basques speak an isolated language which is not related to any surrounding language. This could mean that their unique sounds, words and grammar were totally isolated from other people because of their mountainous environment and climate. It is also conceivable that it is one of the oldest surviving languages, dating to before the arrival of the Indo-Europeans. There is also the Rhaeto-Romanic language of the Alps between Northeastern Italy and Southeastern Switzerland, which has survived until today with a similar condition of being isolated in a steep mountain milieu.

Many original dialects and languages disappeared because of the influences and interactions from outside. Unfortunately many with exotic or extraordinary sounds and signs have died already, and from today's languages only one-tenth will survive the next 100 years. Because the modern world is aware of their uniqueness, many languages are now receiving further protection to keep their exclusivity alive and preserve their culture.

In Central and South America, in the Mazatec language, for example, preserves tonal differences in pitch which represent the meaning of words. Changing one tone distinguishes word meanings and grammatical patterns. This feature is also found in numerous Chinese languages as well as in countries South of the Sahara. Mazatec also has 'whistled speech'–whistles communicated through distances, where normal speech was difficult.

Resemblances among different languages in diverse parts of the world are interesting and tell us about the creativity and human development as adaptation as well as trace their nomadic journeys prior to settlement. Native American languages such as Navajo (see Chapter X) and Apache, for example, belong to the Athabaskan language group, spoken from Alaska to the American Southwest, possibly connected to or migrated from Asia two thousand years ago.

Vowels and pitch characterize languages as well as consonants; imitating rainforest sounds becomes part of language and music. In many languages we find unique sounds, like click-sounds, a sign of interjections or indicators for disapproval. In South African languages these clicks are part of the lyrics as we can hear in the Bantu language; audible in the songs of Miriam Makheba. A language called 'bird-language,' found in Eastern Turkey, uses the chirps and warble sounds of birds. Humans seem to create and adapt to their environment, imitate nature and use sounds coming from the purest sources, using this in music and language. The limitations or extensions of those sounds

---

13. See *Atlas of the Languages* for more detailed information.

are echoed through cultural dependence, language and education.If we realize that half of the world's population is bilingual or multilingual, we can imagine the intensive impact of this on individuals, their creativity and development. In the Netherlands, a Dutch-speaking nation with a multilingual education, four different languages are taught at schools: Dutch, English, French and German. The Dutch are well known for their open-minded worldview and it is possible to think that this is related to their educational model. Another example is people in former colonies, for example, India as a colony of Britain, where three languages are regularly spoken: the local dialect or language of their origin, the official language of the country and probably English, the language of the former empire. Indians, with their 200 indigenous languages, are multilingual because they all learned these at school.

Linguists have shown that being bilingual or multilingual has cognitive advantages and no handicaps. The benefits include an additional openness and acceptance for dissimilar or bizarre sounds, words, senses and expressions. Being familiar with different sounds and experiencing objects as having various names increases the vocabulary of expression, including words, sounds and intonation. Bilingual education is important for cultural integration, understanding differences and enabling communities to learn tolerance. Linguists are convinced that supporting bilingual education will intensify the appreciation of the mother tongue or minority language along with its associated cultural traditions. It also might create at first largely arbitrary meanings and confusion if one object has different names, but finally the benefits compensate for the inconveniences. Bilingually educated young children show that after incomprehension, they benefit from learning other languages in the cultural, communicative, cognitive and emotional aspects of human life.

The emotional impact of language might have the strongest effect at the beginning of learning; it is really hard as an adult to process an unidentified language, listen to outlandish sounds, eccentric word constructions and articulate weird vocal sounds. But with this learning process, a new world of sound, meaning and understanding opens–comparable to listening to different kinds of music. Opening our ears generates emotional space and attention, providing awareness through being subject to indefinite sounds. To learn and become accustomed to more sounds and languages leads to the process of deeper personal discovery and unforeseen contact, teaches tolerance, eases communication and supports self-comfort and self-actualisation.

MY MULTICULTURAL VOICE

Having struggled with different languages, cultures, sounds and music myself, I'd like to share my inner personal process of growth, adapting unusual sounds, words and expressions. Growing up behind the Wall in East Germany–an overprotected, disciplined environment, surrounded by German language and to me the unattractive dialect of my region, Saxony–for years I was a bit ashamed when people recognized my background. Opposing a government that dictated the rules of life like dominant parents formed normal life in East Germany. Father State's demands were systematically forcing an alienation from my own nature and individuality. I lived with feelings of hate and of being totally controlled and curbed, trying to fit in or fulfill the requirements and expectations of this 'fatherly' force (in private the state was called "father state"). Not being able to express my thoughts and opinions openly put pressure on me. Being in conflict with myself in public life, I compensated in my personal life by joking about it. Using humour to make fun of the dominant political ideology lightened the loss of my inner orientation. Luckily my home environment supported and encouraged any form of vocal rebellion; together we made fun about the reality we could not change. I also continued this expression on my own. Naturally that meant unconsciously singing and freely improvising at home during moments of happiness or disappointment to cope with personal aspects or defeat.

The sublime German culture dominated my growth and I discovered its treasures of philosophy, literature and classical music. When I reached the age of travel I started being interested in foreign countries and their cultures to compensate for life behind the Wall. Hungary, Poland, Bulgaria, Romania and Czechoslovakia were the countries I was allowed to visit, practicing my Russian and tiny English vocabulary that I had learned at school. Most people did not like to speak Russian abroad and surprisingly often I could use German or English. But my trips opened my perception to new, unusual sounds, odd smells, colours and different types of people. All were weird and wonderful and mysterious. Searching for a direction in my life, soon I fell in love with the mesmerizing Gypsy and Hungarian folk music, not aware yet that I must have admired the freedom of their vocal and instrumental improvisations and dancing.

I spent time trying out different professions. When I studied classical music professionally in East Germany, I studied to be the perfect performer. Unknowingly I woke up a suppressed need in myself. Through singing I became aware of the powerful capacity of my vocal expression. I pushed and pressured my voice, searching for classical gleaming sounds. I discovered the emotional beauty of the romantic songs of Brahms and Schumann; there was nothing in life so meaningful as singing out what I felt deep inside. Studying Bach in

Leipzig's Gewandhaus choir, I perfected the performance of every nuance of his motifs; singing in this tradition made me rooted in my own culture. Aside from German I tried singing in different tongues. But the beauty decreased when I struggled with the weird pronunciations, winding my lips and tongue into irritating positions. I produced strange, unfamiliar sounds, without being able to feel the deep meaning of the words. I truly hated Russian, Italian and English while I was forced to learn them in language classes; I had not developed any sensitivity for languages and strange sounds in my childhood.

I left my life behind the Wall before the end of the Cold War and moved to the Netherlands. Leaving my home and uncertain if I ever could return, the most critical time of my life started. Every day I felt free of boundaries, but prisoner of my inner limitations. Feeling like a handicapped person, newly adapting to an entirely unknown lifestyle, political system, culture and language, I was truly uncomfortable. Pronouncing words with wrong understanding and attempting new daily rhythms, rules and systems was frustrating. Formulating the same word two, three, four or five times, I felt like an infant learning the simplest steps of life when everybody else already knew them. The Dutch sounds I had to create, pronounced at the back of my throat, did not exist in me; I had not developed those sounds in my life before. Living in the outlandish sounds of another culture is especially different than travelling through it. I felt like an idiot, becoming exhausted about normal things, like getting the right products from the grocery store or making myself understood on the phone.

I coped with this frustration through outbursts of heavy crying, expressing my doubts and regrets. Trying to overcome this I motivated myself through rigorous language study to structure my life again. While life in the Netherlands offered me an unfamiliar personal and political liberty with wonderful opportunities I intensely enjoyed, I was beaten by culture shock.

Still searching for unrestricted freedom in sound, I sang and screamed in a pop band while I was studying music therapy in Nijmegen (NL). I also reconnected myself to my German roots performing songs of Kurt Weill and discovering the unknown persona of popular music in myself. Through the years I established a new personality: from an East German speaking an unattractive Saxony dialect, I grew in to a throaty Dutch-speaking person singing any musical style. After mastery of this, the need to improve my English grew. Irritated and unable to have conversations with the world, I travelled to Malta, a bilingual island, to study for the first time in my life real English language. I felt that the quality of my life improved through discovering the world with new ears and tongues; the variety of sounds expanded my reality and perhaps my personality. Finally getting comfortable speaking English, I was excited to 'contact the world.' I experienced the liberation of not hiding my limited language skills anymore and wanted to communicate with everyone. I was content to switch from English to Dutch or German. People told me years later that whenever I switched languages they experienced my personality shift. I believe that the process of growing through unfamiliar, frightening sounds and being uncomfortable with our own limitations is like moving through a long dark tunnel. The various languages and sounds had made a particular impact on me, reassuring my self-esteem. But there were more remarkable aspects to discover.

The knowledge about the natural capacity of my vocal sounds arose when I started voicework, exploring my natural voice. Singing classical let me feel that there was nothing more beautiful to express; exploring my natural voice with fascinating sounds let me reach the deepest hidden levels of my personality. And for the first time I felt that I could liberate my whole personality and that I had found parts of my own authentic voice. Pleasurably expressing any possible sound helped clean up many frustrations and difficulties I had assembled. I lost the shame of my background and its limitations, accepting the shadow parts of myself through becoming vocally and emotionally united. While working intensively through bodywork, I surprised myself with emotional sounds escaping my body. Mirroring my new authentic sounds I met bizarre ones, female as well as male in character. I wondered, was there also a man inside of me?

The next step in my life brought me to Turkey; life in this outlandish culture did not truly confuse me anymore–no new culture shock. Now I was experienced, my expectations had become more realistic but still I was learning to cope with unforeseen eccentric sounds and moments. Listening to Sufi music and practicing oriental scales and songs in the Turkish language, and sharing life with the community in Istanbul, finally became a routine and calmed me. The microtones in Middle Eastern scales appeared as extremely delicate forms of emotions to me and conveyed new vocal sensations, deeply touching me and easily moving me to or away from tears. I never consciously experienced microtones in my voice before, but I realized their impact on me was to give me an emotional regulator. I used to make microtonal sounds through creating vibratos; but now those microtones come out of me organically, sounding out those feelings I did not know about. I was astonished; was my soul singing, too?

The world of unusual sound opened me again to additional insight. I felt that my way of singing softened up; I became more feminine, more sensitive, affected by the rich variations of Middle Eastern music and its improvisations. The spiritual aspect of singing was new for me and I did not understand it. The subtle vibration of the microtones affected my body and mind and it seemed to me that the waves of sound could penetrate the cosmos–wherever that might be. Being adaptive to my environment and reflective to my inner potential, I practiced trance. I repeatedly experienced different stages of consciousness through singing for myself during shamanistic exercises. Curious and fearful that I had entered unknown territory, I trained myself to sing in a structured way. Soon I recognized that the vibration of my sounds affected my whole body, softly shaking it repeatedly, and my simplest understanding of this was a profound experience of resonance. I was able to relax deeply and my mind wandered into guided directions, the entrance of different levels of consciousness, moments of trance. Practicing those techniques I became familiar with trance and discovered the depth of this through exceptionally personal experiences. I believe that I became able to communicate with the most buried parts of my Self and evocated the anxiety that appeared.

Changing cultures again, the door to more sounds and bewilderment opened: studying music therapy in advanced master program in the US. I had already practiced music therapy for years, but doing so in the English language was different from the professional world I knew. It was in New York, where I was mature enough to seriously share my experiences and mixture of sounds for the first time in life. Again struggling with weird expressions, verbal limitations and confusion as every foreigner in New York does, I kept searching for my own authentic voice. While I was exposed to additional languages, peculiar sounds and fast food, I needed to ground myself in my own cultural context. Having advanced myself through the many adaptations and countless misunderstandings I had undergone through the years, I kept my voice trained and my eyes and ears attentive. I met an authentic American voice during a voice workshop, which delightfully contacted and communicated with me. From this sudden voice connection I developed a personal and professional relationship with Kate Richards Geller. We sang with each other for years before developing our voice-training workshop, "A Time To Sing." And finally I desired to write this book, processing consciously my personal and professional development. Only after the many years of developing my myriad inner voices, and then experiencing the enormous support of the New York City community, was I ready to express my own 'Authentic Voice.'

THE FOREIGN VOICE – A CASE EXAMPLE

During one of the many trips to Turkey, I experienced a remarkable vocal harmony while connected with a little 4- or 5-year-old girl whom I'll call Media. Understanding no Turkish or Kurdish language spoken in this environment, I communicated vocally with Media, connecting and bonding myself through our universal voices, overcoming her fear and isolation.

Visiting an Island in the Sea of Marmara, close to Istanbul, I got in contact with a Kurdish family living in a tiny house surrounded by a big garden. Travelling with my friend who had met this family before, as we entered their garden, the family warned us of their daughter's strange reaction. No danger was expected from her but an exhausting outburst of crying when Media saw strangers. The family was annoyed and ashamed of her reaction, wrongly interpreting her behaviour as unwelcoming of visitors. To prevent those crises, the family did not introduce Media to strangers but kept her in the house throughout visits. During conversation in the garden with the family, whose Kurdish my friend translated, the mother mentioned more about the problems of her daughter, getting comfortable after she learned that I was a therapist. She told us that whenever Media would see a visitor or stranger who was not a direct family member, she would break into tears. Once she started crying, nobody and nothing could stop her for hours. She seemed to be overwhelmed by visitors' voices: their sudden appearance and warm but insensitive welcome. Unable to cope with the effect of it, her only reaction was an intense outburst of crying to express her distress. Media's mother, unable to stop the crying, was desperate for help or advice in this isolated part of Istanbul.

I was curious and comfortable when the mother asked me if I could see her daughter. Believing in the unique transformation of the girl's emotions into sound and in my experience through vocal work with other children during their outbursts, I was prepared for whatever would happen. When the mother opened the door to the house we lowered our voices, waiting for the moment the girl would notice us and start crying. When Media appeared in the door, we all stopped talking. Slowly she turned her face into a searching movement, shoved her body along the door, looked around, not directly into our faces–but did not cry. Thinking of autistic behaviour I decidedly gave her time to discover the situation, to create a form of safety by refraining from welcoming her heartily as all visitors had done before.

Keeping a safe distance, extremely softly I started talking to Media in my language, kneeling down and saying her name. No crying. I was sure that I used wrong pronunciations of her name, but I communicated with her in any language but Kurdish. Aware of this I started to switch from talking to simply using exhales, making sound and finally humming musically to ease our conversation. No crying. While I intensified my humming into singing I moved closer to Media, keeping a simple ostinato pattern. No crying. I honestly became disenchanted because I had prepared to sing along with her crying. When I later tried to introduce soft hand clapping as a musical way of making contact and creating a rhythmic structural pattern, Media, instead of crying or turning away, took my hand and pulled me away from the family. Surprised by her action and being aware of her mother's observation, I let the little girl pull me through the garden. Curious about her plans and the intensity of her directions, I followed her. Media walked with me out of the garden, down the empty street while she was holding my hand. I continuously supported our walk and sang to her simple patterns of repetitive short melodies, exchanging and mirroring her sounds, clapping our hands and creating primitive songs like improvised lullabies.

It was a peaceful summer day I never will forget: being a stranger on this island, city and country, not knowing language and direction, I was comfortable communicating with Media in her home environment, listening to singing birds, humming and singing in various sounds and any language we produced, and responding to the sounds around us. I felt we were creating a matchless isolated language of whistles and bizarre sounds, communicating like birds or other animals, using no words. I realized that this girl was able to listen and interact with my sounds, which were foreign to her but adapted to her environment. It seemed to be easier for Media to communicate nonverbally with me than with her own culture. This vocal interchange seemed to me intensely reassuring, rooting us in the earliest tradition of human communication. Despite the difference in our backgrounds, education level, culture, language, and oral and musical tradition, we shared an archetypical understanding of ourselves and our environment. Our multicultural conversation was so natural; it was as if we understood our differences, and that such understanding enabled us to communicate tolerance.

When I turned back to her home, Media had difficulties accepting this change in direction. Singing simple melodies and clapping hands in a playful way I encouraged her moving back. While offering rhythmical structure I waited and respected the moments she needed for adjustment. Finally she followed my offer, walking back without crisis or crying. During the 15 to 20 minutes of our vocal, emotional and musical contact, Media cooperated wonderfully. When we entered the garden her mother was waiting, and she was thrilled by what she had witnessed. She told us that her daughter never was able to go away with somebody, never was so cooperative and always cried when seeing visitors. I helped her understand the situation, mentioning that I was communicating and comforting her daughter through sensitive sounds like humming and singing. I encouraged the mother to sing herself and suggested that this could comfort her daughter in her fears and panic attacks or even could prevent them. Laughing regretfully, the mother admitted that she could not sing. Understanding the transcultural value of the paralinguistic expression I just had experienced with the girl, I hoped that her mother was rooted in the same traditional existence. But she was not; singing did not belong to her reality and she seemed unable to adapt my suggestions. Sadly I acknowledged that the mother was far away from understanding her daughter's acoustic symbols, her individual needs and emotional contact. But how could this woman understand the need of her handicapped and I would guess stimulatory-sensory deprived child? I, as a therapist, knew that the vocal unity we just had developed was unique and transcended cultural barriers. This exchange of our individual expressions could possibly translate into more growth if I could stay for longer. Thankful for this extraordinary experience, somewhat delighted but troubled that I could not offer more help, we departed. I still remember that beautiful summer day, thinking of this beautiful girl Media. Does she still cry, or did she find someone who could adapt her unusual sounds into an emotional, multicultural or universal understanding? And was her overwhelming environment developing the sensitivity to bridge into her isolated sounds and communicate with her?

Chapter V

My search for understanding spirituality and vocal expression as transmitter into different stages of consciousness and trance is the content of this chapter. In *Spiritual Voices* I explain how our world and culture is changing and how we are moving from one worldview to another. Following Ken Wilber's interpretation of the world and illumination, singing in a spiritual context attunes us to the universe so that we can be sensitive and sympathetic toward all levels of experience–and also to the unknown 'whispering voices.' *Trance Voices* explains Adam Crabtree's daily switches into different states of consciousness as well as the effects of the intense vibration of vocal sound. *My Transcending Voice* describes my personal trance experiences through structured singing in shamanistic form and explains differences between traditional shamanistic rituals and structured singing. *The Grieving Voice* details an example of trance-like singing in a mourning ritual with a girl in a special education program.

SPIRITUAL VOICES

Inquisitive about explanations of spirituality, willing to accept the existence of different levels of consciousness, I searched for an interpretation of my personal experiences. To sing and resonate with another meant to me being emphatically connected. Singing together with Kate Richards Geller offered us both totally new occurrences: dialoguing with our voices we were sharing a 'common world-space' with each other, as Wilber called it. During our singing we shared a basic emotional space that embraced everything from the core physical level to the highest level of our spiritual consciousness. Our communicating voices would bridge into the air, the universe or just into the open space of our human existence, exchanging messages.

The woman who was screaming during my accident with the van (described in Chapter II) was sharing the basic emotion with me, too. Through her empathic resonance she sent out an instinctive call as a warning of danger. This common context of sharing the emotional place in the world permits the interpretation of empathic resonance with each other. We all can be connected to this lower world space, the physical or gravitational power, the vegetative or the reptilian, animalistic level of life we share. We can communicate with animals and be certain that they understand us. And we can make instinctive or animalistic sounds to exchange information. But we share more: we also contain complex cognitive, theoretical and linguistic backgrounds. And we position our shared interpretations in these common cultural backgrounds.

So complex are our shared backgrounds, our communication patterns are changing and with them our contexts. Our place in the world and our cultures are changing, we are moving from one worldview to another: from archaic to magical to mythical to rational to existential (Wilber). Today we are at a higher, integral vantage point from to see all these worldviews and interpret the cosmos[14], analysing both psychology and religion. Moving through different stages of human life seems to be common, but we are not as easily conscious about moving in a cosmic order. This becomes pertinent when we discuss trance and shamanistic voices, as in the following sections of this book. We need to be aware that everything we do affects the bigger picture. Every step of movement or progress includes a small change in our minds and possibly a giant transformation in history. Letting go of old interpretations and preparing for new ones, expecting and accepting change, making progress–these processes are similar in personal and collective life.

Focused on singing, I expect to gain a deeper understanding of the interpretations of the cosmos. In my search, I consider the phenomena of sound and especially the sound of voices. Sound is a physical vibration within a context of time and space. My dictionary offers me 24 explanations of sound. Which one is correct depends on context and my personal interpretation. From the 24 I chose my context for sound as 'the particular auditory effect produced by a given cause.' I interpret that the cause could be the vibration of vocal cords of a voice. The energy concept of Pythagoras taught us that anything that moves or vibrates is giving a sound. Every movement in nature–the sun, the moon, the trees of the earth and of course human beings–causes vibrations of different frequencies. These frequencies are measurable and many descriptions of natural sounds are available. For example, in the books of Joachim-Ernst Berendt, *The World is Sound* and *The Third Ear*, many interpretations of sound are described. Berendt concentrates on the importance of listening to nature and the world. He has countless examples of frequencies of natural sources. He compares nature's sound and the environmental perception through the ear, with the usual 'tele'-focused function of the eyes in our society. It was interesting for me to learn that in the Greek language 'tele' means 'distant' or 'end' and television, for example, makes the connections between distant objects. Behrendt brings awareness of the ear in to our television-eye-oriented society. With this ear-oriented sounding awareness, he pictures the importance not of distance, but rather of closeness and attachment through sound. The voice is the best connector to closeness and attachment through sounding awareness and personal contact.

14. The common interpretation of the word cosmos is 'order'; or the world or universe regarded as an orderly, harmonious system (Stein, 1966, *The Random Dictionary*).

I'd like to stay with the voice as the source of sound and to portray a very simple interpretation of it: I sing out into the world. Look at Appendix C about the vibration of a human vowel with its structured design. This sound makes an auditory effect and vibrates from my body into the environment. It touches other material or humans and vibrates and eventually resonates with them. Through this resonance the sound becomes stronger and penetrates into the nature of a special culture or environment and receives waves of understanding. The context of the sound can be a meaningful vocal expression, which resonates in somebody else's voice and body and becomes encouraged to vibrate more because of that understanding. This process can be a deep personal experience, resonating with people in the same emotional space. This can be a vocal experience between Kate and me, resonating in a common world-space. But can my song also be heard in a different place in the world because we also contain complex cognitive, theoretical and linguistic backgrounds? And can we transcend physical boundaries and travel great distances just by our intention? What is a spiritual experience? Can the singing voice of a person vocalize a prayer and vibrate into the universe? Can these sounds be heard, held and understood through the emphatic resonance of nature, the cosmos or believers in God practicing ritual? Are there archetypes that we conjure up through a singing ritual that connect us to faraway cultures even when there is no intention?

Wilber makes the point that we can and do interpret the world in a variety of ways. The way in which we interpret the world and our experiences is with "illumination." Thus the way we illuminate our experiences is the way we share ourselves with the world, the way our interpretation streams with our own self-system, and the way we communicate about it with others. I interpreted sound as described above and I searched for people who experienced and understood sound of a voice with similar illumination. Kate, for example, communicated, understood and shared my illuminated experience through her own interpretation; perhaps she connected herself to faraway cultures even without intention, or she practiced a ritual.

But we share more and we continue exploring the phenomenon illuminated interpretation often not knowing what it means. Our own extraordinary depth escapes us, confuses us and through our misinterpretation we obscure the truth, because we cannot interpret it adequately.

It requires great subtlety to find the exact interpretation for those deeper experiences and sensations of human life. If we acknowledge that the basic rule of interpretation is its context, then we have something to grasp. We need to reassure ourselves that we test our interpretations and see if they fit into the larger context. This means focusing on many levels of experience, the material, physical, mental and spiritual ones by noticing, analysing, and comparing them before we determine their meaning. Excluding different emphases on the material, body, mind or spirit is limiting our personal and collective interpretations as worldviews have done.

Many worldviews overlook the variation of these levels of experience and miss the whole truth. In New Age philosophy, for example, a reaction to pragmatic developments in the West, concentrates chiefly on one aspect: the development of the higher Self, or consciousness, and neglects the rational and the behavioral aspects, and denies or repressed the ego (especially the shadow). Other worldviews focus mainly on the collective side such as the socialistic, communistic society I grew up in, and lose sight of the uniqueness of the individual. After I left my homeland I needed to work on my very individual development and my responsibility for my own worldview. People of former East Germany still suffer from the need for individual responsibility after being accustomed to 40 years of collective care. It is significant to understand that we all personally and collectively prioritize life with different emphases on the material, body, mind or spirit. Merely by experiencing materialistic, physical, mental and spiritual processes and moving fruitfully through each of these developmental levels, we create a healthy sense of identity. Only through those productive movements of experience can an identity transcend its limits and develop a form of harmony. Higher or deeper stages of consciousness can be reached only through the human process of growth and development. We all carry so much resistance, but through experiencing these levels, various forms of truthfulness, can unfold. We need to attune ourselves to the universe to be sensitive and sympathetic toward all levels of experience[15]. Personally, we move from one developmental level to another and collectively, we release ourselves to other, more inclusive worldviews, as we search for authentic transformation.

This cosmic attunement is essential for therapeutic work as well as for teaching. To attain deep resonance with our clients and students requires listening to these different levels, sensations and sounds of life. Besides focusing on our own priorities, we have to keep our ears open for sounds of every possible utterance to develop spiritual intuition. Wilber describes the sympathetic attunement with all aspects of the cosmos as being different voices we need to listen to and to interpret correctly in order to continue moving to higher levels of understanding.

---

15. I remember how deeply I was touched by a special group of dancing dervishes, an unusual mix of men and women in multicolored dresses in an original Sufi place in Istanbul. I realized that there must be something more than I knew about dance and transformation. Seeing men and woman through dance and music connected into trance in an Islamic society brought my tears up. Personally experiencing strongly the split between male and female in this culture, I was touched by this spiritual unity. There must exist other forms of connection that I never experienced, a deep rooting to spirituality or contact with God and the cosmos where the difference between men and woman, poor and rich, have disappeared.

> And we begin to do so by noticing that each speaks to us with a different voice. If we listen carefully, we can hear each of these voices whispering gently their truths, and finally joining in a harmonious chorus that quietly calls us home. . . . But we must listen very carefully. (104)

Achieving harmony sounds cliché, but listening to every possible uttered voice as a means of integration of oneself with the cosmos is a profound process for those who wish to develop a sensitive, personal and professional attitude. Listening and analysing voices while processing materialistic, physical and mental levels of development actually bring us closer to the interpretation of spiritual experiences.

TRANCE VOICES

Vibrations of voices and whispers can be heard and perceived in spiritual moments of trance as well as in coma, as I will explain later, fostered through singing or listening to music. I'd like to describe a trance technique that is a structured form of singing with intention, concentration and purpose, without an audience. This is different from the trance-like moments that can happen when one is singing unconsciously, as when cleaning the basement, or concentrated singing, as when rehearsing in a choir. Crabtree (1997) differentiates trance as a natural part of everyday existence and reminds me that we live and experience a "tapestry of trance states," unaware that we are switching from one into another. Acknowledging that trance is also a natural if repressed experience in Western cultures, it is crucial to explain that trance cannot be made to happen, but will suddenly arise from one moment to the next. In the following section I will focus on what kind of spiritual or bodily sensations are present and what tangibly happens during intentional structured singing with awareness.

I believe that when we are singing with intention in a structured way, repeating two tones in a simple repetitive rhythm like an ostinato or centric melody (for instance a tonic and a third), we can entirely live out the sound by accessing the hidden potentials available in sound. We can bring our bodies to a stage of physical relief: a full and deep experience of resonance, a deep vibration of tones. Sokolov points out in her "embodied voicework" that after repeated deep breathing exercises, one may have the sensation of opening the muscles of the body; finally the whole body is breathing and making the sound, not just the throat and mouth. When the entire body is integrated in this process, the totality of vibration can cause relief for "the internal system of the body." This strong, energetic form of vibration occurs in individual parts, as well as in the body as a whole, on cellular, muscular and neurological levels (see Chapter VI). This vibration is energetic and is connected through waves that the sound is sending out. It creates organized forms and patterns, as shown in the picture in Appendix C, which vibrate inside and outside of the body. The energy source is pure, physical, wave vibration. Vibrations of the waves bring the cells into periodic motion. These vibrations create different frequencies in the body. Through these frequencies, the body is mobilized: shaken through tiny, wave-like movements through the whole body and involving each cell of the entire system. In this heightened state, the 'old' regions of the brain are activated (see Chapter VI), evoking archetypes of nature that are part of collective unconscious. These archetypes emerge in the early moments of the trance experience; from here, the individual can travel deeper into intense dreams or ecstasy. Boundaries between these states are malleable.

In daily life we are able to switch from one state of consciousness to another: from an everyday world, 'here and now' orientation to a deeper knowledge, a super-personal wisdom; a.k.a., 'higher consciousness,' which helps us to grasp what is not yet clear or conscious. In the everyday world we can slide spontaneously in and out of the subconsciousness of a daydream and the twilight moments just before we wake up or fall asleep. From this subconscious state, we enter into different states of consciousness easily.

Through vibrato, those different states of consciousness can be intensified: the brain can be triggered as in the condition of deep meditation and creative moments (see Chapter VI). Also, the heart and blood pressure can be regulated because of the sympathetic vibration of the skeleton. Through vocal training, the brilliance of overtones[16] can be felt in some body parts. These overtone frequencies can create a tiny new organization and structure within the body, which vibrates and moves, loosening and liberating cells and muscles, stimulating body liquids and muscular coordination. Relaxation or extension of old forms within the body can help remove any blockage and stimulate greater vibration, which can support a change in frozen, inflexible parts in the body. Emotional shocks, bodily injuries, traumas and accidents can create many kinds of physical and psychological blocks. When a physical block is diffused or removed and the body is stimulated to follow the natural flow of energy, the body's internal systems are activated and the immune system will improve. I believe that all healing is ultimately self-healing, activating the physical and mental capacity toward well-being and health. Through moments of trance those capacities can be attained.

With both structured singing and with the shamanistic tradition (archaic series of techniques to achieve non-ordinary states of awareness; a kind of

16. Overtones are higher harmonic tones that are mathematically related to the fundamental tone or frequency.

ecstasy), music and vocal sounds are used to memorize the route to achieve the altered state of consciousness, characterized by a heightened, detached state. In traditional shamanism, the healing power comes from outside the individual through a connection with the power of nature and its spirits. During a form of structured singing without a shaman, I experienced healing from inside through a connection with the personal power of the individual–with my Self[17]. This is related to traditional approaches where the self-healing capacity of the voice is stimulated without help from outside.

In traditional shamanistic rituals, the voice is the connector and awakener of the animal spirits and the drum is the transporter for the traveler. The shaman recites, chants, screams or sings words and melodies to the spirits and invokes their power. A shaman is able to awaken the power, which is different from the personal power of structured singing I describe. I use a shamanistic structure during my singing but not its traditional power because I am not a shaman. Both forms, the shamanistic tradition and the structured singing, follow the same purpose of passing boundaries and transcending into spiritual states of consciousness, a careful shifting from one state to another. In shamanism and singing there are general, analogous levels for this process of traveling to a spiritual state. One major difference between the two is the role of the traveler: In shamanism, the shaman travels, connecting with the spirits. It is he who gets into the trance and takes his client with him. During structured singing, it is the person him- or herself who gets into trance. In Part B of this book I will describe more about shamanistic traditions. For now I would like to describe the process of travelling and accessing a deep trance through structured singing.

The process of travelling to a spiritual state through structured singing requires four steps. The first could be seen as awareness, meaning an emotional, physical and environmental preparation for the process: silence in the room, sitting or lying comfortably, concentrating attention. Second is the actualization of material and relaxation of the traveler: what kind of vocal sounds, pitch, duration, pattern, melody or words get initiated, intensified and repeated. The third step is the journey, the state of trance–the ecstatic condition in an altered state of consciousness. This step requires the use of vocal sound to help the traveler adapt, intensify, change or stay firm as s/he moves through the trance

---

17. I am not a trained shaman and will not describe any shamanistic rituals. I was supported by a shamanistically trained psychologist, and followed books such as *Secrets of Shamanism*, a good guide during my self-training. I also need to stress the importance of guides. Books are helpful but a personal guide can reconnect or stop the trance if the experience is too intense. It is better not to go into deep trance without training, knowledge or experience of it. There are various techniques for travel into trance; it is possible without the use of the voice, for example, by listening to certain relaxing music or drumming. I personally prefer the voice because of the vibratory connection with body and mind.

imagery. The last step is the re-entry, meaning the integration, reflection and the activity of returning to the normal state of consciousness, involving a decrease in vocal sound, deep relaxation, orientation to here-and-now and awareness of silence in the room.

The longest and most important element of this process is the third step, the experience of trance. Often a trance is characterized by images of nature and archetypical visualizations: passages, trails and bridges, mountains, bodies of water, birds, especially the eagle, specific animals or animal imagery, such as unicorns, bears, wolves and tigers. A symbolic connection to the inner world of the traveler is always made through the animals, the residents of nature. Archetypical functions bridge the different worlds: flying, walking, swimming or riding to the upper, middle, under, and normal worlds. These worlds are remarkable levels of consciousness made accessible through singing in the trance state. In this state the imagination can be visual and auditory, and can even bring physical body sensations.

During structured singing I experience the voice as the guide that connects the body and mind. It is easy to shift into deeper connections where "the cosmos sings through their voices and the spirit shines through their eyes," as Wilber poetically describes. Through singing into this connection, different worlds are accessible to the trance traveler. During these intense vocal sounds, my entire body experiences the acoustic sound as a personal identification with the subjects to whom I am connecting, whether patients or peers.

I learned from Wilber that consciousness, depth and spirit are synonymous. Depth swells from the subconscious, the daydream from the self-conscious, and self-knowledge from the superconscious, the cosmic awareness. Receiving the simple benefits of consciousness exploration is possible for anyone, resulting in states of consciousness rising to a light or deep state of trance[18]. Trance-like states initiated through a singing ritual can form a bridge to an altered state of consciousness in vocal music therapy. Trance has been used for centuries and in every culture this practice has always had the purpose of self-healing, whether through intentional rituals or unconscious effect. There is no need to exclude this phenomenon as something belonging to other cultures.[19]

---

18. To enter the superconscious requires long training, advanced techniques, in-depth processing, and the intention for higher personal development, as required for the shaman.

19. I met David Lewiston, a British specialist of world music recordings and documentations, when both of us were in Istanbul, Turkey. He told me that his goal of making quality recordings of world music was to "share the beauty of it." He said that some of this music was transporting him to "deep peaceful inner space". He wrote in *Voices of Forgotten Worlds* about his appreciation for trance states: "I still don't understand trance, it's still a very great mystery, but my travels have made me realize that spirit possession is by no means uncommon. It exists, for example, throughout the Himalayas and Karakorams, and the islands of Indonesia. . . . Ever since I witnessed these rites I've come to accept that there is another world, the world of spirits, invisible, intangible, but very real all the same." (p. 9).

Our sensitivity to sonic information means that everybody, independent of their tradition and culture, can learn to receive and understand vibration, and to connect themselves to spiritual, magical states or moments of trance.

MY TRANSCENDING VOICE

While I was having countless clinical and non-clinical trance-like experiences, I decided to practice shamanistic exercises in Turkey to seriously discover and explore the power of my personal singing. I wrote about my personal trance experiences, concentrating on what happens to me during a deep, self-induced form of trance. I'd like to describe how I personally experienced my vibrating voice in a trance to relax and heal myself.

Describing my personal trance training, I will use my private images and experiences to give examples of the diversity of traveling practice. Always preparing myself for the intense impact of the trance and the time I need to readjust, I set a time limit of two or three hours, removing the telephone and other interruptions in the room. Starting in a relaxed position of lying or sitting with closed eyes, I bring my breath to a simple balanced exchange of inhale and exhale. Minutes later I utter a low vocal sound, comfortable for my voice, around "G" or "F," letting this sound vibrate through my body and develop into a rhythmical form which I easily can repeat. After a while, the vowel and rhythm begin to sing themselves and they change naturally, adjusting to the most comfortable pattern that I can sing on one exhale, finally without effort or conscious awareness. Continuing that pattern, the sound travels through my body, vibrating and loosening tension, and I guide myself to favourite places in nature. I travel to a well-known beach where a little fire is burning or to a small path through green woods, waiting for pictures and images to appear. During my early trance state, I often see an eagle, panther, turtle or a curiously shaped fish. Those animals, which regularly come to me, carry important symbolic meanings for me, which I learned later through interpretations in shamanistic books.

When my self-induced trance moves to a deeper level through the repetition of vocal sound and its intense vibrations, relaxing and focusing me on images, it is time to make contact with the animals. Asking important personal questions, questions of life, problems of the moment, or sometimes just my sense of curiosity brings up imaginary conversation with these animals. While asking at those moments for help with personal issues, it is important not to push myself to intellectual, "linear" thinking, since trying to control the situation could make me suddenly come out of the trance. I stay focused on my sound, correct my posture if needed, intensify my focus on the images that appear, and allow the feelings of relaxation to gradually broaden my perception. My receptivity for ideas, pictures or images is intensified in deep state of trance and often surprises me with 'answers.' Touching the source of human creativity or universal wisdom, I feel that I am attuning myself to the cosmos, communicating with "one of those whispering voices."

During my early trance experience, besides my well-known animals, often a spider would appear, walking through the picture of my imagination. Annoyed by this creature (unpleasant for me), I noticed my mind trying to push it away. But often it would come back, and after weeks of training I became aware of its significance. Being unaware about the vibrations my body sent out, I understood that my cells and muscles had touched a deep level of angst in me and brought it into physical and emotional awareness. Identifying the spider as a filtered picture of unconscious fear, I was able to get in touch with it. Having always been afraid of spiders and their unpredictable behaviour, I finally understood my avoidance of them.

Intensifying my vocal sounds while in trance made me feel stronger, more grounded and better prepared to face this fear taking form through a moving, uncontrollable spider. Through the relaxed state of trance, a safer, more detached perspective towards this fear was possible. Gradually, I dared to look at the spider, and it was horrifying to me. Watching the insect, I became shocked when it grew bigger and moved around uncontrollably. But I continued my sound and did not interrupt my trance. I knew through my training that I could stop when the fear overwhelmed me–different from dreams (with the exception of lucid dreams), where no conscious interventions are normally possible. But my sound let me get in contact with myself and I was able to transcend physical and emotional boundaries.

The initial moment of shock when looking at the spider made me feel very small, experiencing existential fear. But suddenly the spider got smaller, too. From this moment I experienced the spider as less dangerous but still capable of changing unpredictable. When I changed my posture, breath or voice, while still keeping the repetitive vocal pattern alive, my inner imagery changed. I realized that I could manipulate the pictures and handle the spider if I did not experience myself as too 'small.' Watching the picture of the spider changing, I slowly dared to play with it and allowed more dynamic changes to happen. Surprisingly, out of one big scary spider many little spiders emerged, walking around like ants but in a controlled and ordered manner. Being aware of this wilful transformation, my fear diminished and a new order and control entered my trance experience.

Finally I decided to end the trance. I walked back the same imaginary pathway through nature and came back to the room I was sitting in and ended my singing. Combined with first gentle, then intensive breath and body movements I woke up my entire body, slowly opening my eyes and lastly orienting myself in the room. Glad to be back in the here and now, my meeting with the spider now receded into a dreamy vagueness. While I took time to return to a normal state of consciousness, I realized the depth of my travel: I had communicated with my subconscious. I had dared to look at the spider for the first time in my life, and came away from the encounter more confident and sure of myself.

This first contact with the spider encouraged me to remain open to communication with this insect in trance experiences that followed. During subsequent contact I sometimes felt physical reactions of nausea, cold or warm rushes or bodily tension. I learned how beneficial the symbol of the spider was for me, and at last I resolved to work on my fear in many of my succeeding trance experiences. While the spider was walking over me or entering every opening of my body, my fear of being out of control was powerfully symbolized through her fast movement. During many following spider-trances I played with my fearful imaginations and finally worked out my existential angst. Personal issues in different areas of my life were evoked by this insect, and I gradually learned to respect the wisdom it represented. After years of unconscious anxiety symbolized by spiders, I could see and tolerate their existence–no need to hysterically scream or run away by facing them.

Often spiders or other insects are seen as repulsive or 'awe-full,' mirroring behaviour, instincts and patterns of archetypical forces we do not fully understand. Shamanistic wisdom opened my sympathy to natural resources and I could illuminate the symbol of the spider as my totem and how it was creating and weaving my fate. The spider symbol helps establish balance between past and future, physical and spiritual, male and female, and I found myself surrendering to all of these poles. This encounter especially focused me on my own personal creativity: as a teacher and a writer, the spider made me aware of my wisdom and creative potential, and I became willing not to follow others anymore. My own creativity was waiting in the dark in more inaccessible areas of my unconscious–just like the spider lives in dark corners. Finally, words formed a creative web as I started writing this book, weaving together my dreams, imaginations, fears and years of experiences.

THE GRIEVING VOICE – A CASE EXAMPLE

In my work with children with special needs, I had the pleasure to work with a 12-year-old girl who touched me profoundly during our musical contact. Shelly is an African-American girl with normal speech development, a high cognitive capacity but with constantly changing moods, often sad and prone to episodic irritability–symptoms of a depressive personality. Since years she lived in a foster home with an elderly woman in her seventies, who she called 'mammy.'

When I met this lady, she would talk to me about Shelly, treating her like a 'retarded' child. Any attempt I made to show her Shelly's high level of development, failed. It seemed that she did not receive the emotional care she needed at home. Her former teacher asked me to take Shelly to the music session to "make her smile" and to give her an outlet for her emotions. Acknowledging that I could not necessarily make her smile, I focused on her depression and seriously addressed her sad feelings. I worked with her individually every week for three and a half years during which time, in fact, she often did smile. Attuning to her needs, I nurtured and in a sense re-parented her.

At the beginning of music therapy Shelly did not talk freely, appearing shy and serious as she did in her classroom, where she was the only girl. Whenever I sang about her playing different instruments, I discovered that she smiled and actively played along with the musical changes. Shelly emerged as extremely musical, and whenever we played any kind of instrument together, her mood and facial expression changed visibly. She said she was 'happy' when she made music. She was able to show a wonderful, authentic smile and move her whole body to the rhythm of the music. She became intensely involved in the music making, played instruments with great coordination, and exhibited significant auditory-motor and sensory-motor skills. She revealed a capacity to create beautiful music, either by following my music or composing her own sounds. Her musicality touched me with its purity and quality. She was very vulnerable and delicate in expressing herself. I was sensing how she took risks when she was playing; her love of music and development of trust seemed to allow her to participate more fully. She benefited mostly from our nonverbal and intense musical interactions and the experience appeared to gradually strengthen her self-esteem, but she was only able to translate a portion of this into daily life. Shelly remained distressed in the classroom, and she never talked positively about herself; whenever I sang something positive about her she looked ashamed or would soon stop me. When she moved to a different classroom, I was able to share my observations about her with her wonderful teacher and build a successful collaboration.

In a later stage of the therapy process, Shelly loved to sit close to me at the piano, choosing and singing 'happy' songs, always avoiding 'sad' music. Any gloomy musical sounds I brought in would be rejected immediately. Rapport developed between us as she asked me to sing for her, and sometimes she joined me vocally for moments during a children's song, repeating my words. She would not dare to sing alone; expressing herself freely through her voice did not seem possible without my support and encouragement.

Last year she changed to a new foster home with a friendlier environment and a younger, caring mother. Shortly after this, Shelly received heartbreaking news from her brother, the only family member she had, that their biological mother had died. She did not participate in any funeral or grieving ceremony. Feeling helpless, miserable and alone without any supportive environment, Shelly had a tough time digesting the changes in her life. She regressed; her depression returned and mood swings increased. During this time she loved playing the keyboard and searched through many kinds of sounds, unconsciously testing which would be closest to her feelings. Still, she avoided dark or sad sounds, unconsciously protecting herself from a profound emotional collapse. While playing long improvisations she appeared to be absorbed in her own sound, musically weaving a cover of comfort for herself. Her playing was mostly very sincere, only occasionally harsh. While playing different instruments, Shelly would never get deeper into her real emotions. We had long musical conversations and built up a nonverbal understanding of each other; this became the basis of our trustworthy contact. In truth I experienced our long play together as merging of communication in a different world-space. She was able to touch sounds in a depth of spirituality and musicality that I had never experienced with another child. After our playing and singing, we always needed time to readjust ourselves to our environment, like coming out of a dream or a deeper form of contact. We took some minutes of silence, observed each other's facial reaction and did not rush back to her classroom.

At the beginning of the new school year Shelly was exceptionally glad to be back to our music routine after the long vacation. It seemed to me as if she felt safe with me to open herself more and tell me about herself, her new home and the absence of her biological mother. She expressed intimate needs and engaged me in young children's games, and she put her head on my shoulder or lap while we were singing. She regressed to a younger developmental stage to nurture and heal her past. She seemed to discover me as a person, using me as a mirror: touching my hands and arms, wondering why my "light" skin was different from hers, or asking me personal questions. She told me that I was her "mammy" or she asked me why I could not be her mother. I realized that I had become her transitional mother figure; she made up the intimacy she had missed in her early years when her mother got sick and disappeared out of her life. Being allowed to act silly as well as challenging me, she tested my reactions like children do with their parents. Her intimate physical needs and playful interactions developed into a wonderful contact. Cooperating with the classroom teacher, acknowledging Shelly's emotional needs, and building on the book she made about her mother, I decided to work for the next months on her grief and loss. I offered a safe place to express and process those feelings as well explore her pleasure in music.

Shelly was curious to know if my mother was still alive and she started talking about her mother and even sometimes about her deep feelings of loss. I decided to address those feelings even though Shelly had avoided touching them in the past. Suddenly she wanted to make a 'happy song' about her mother, but she could not sing by herself and waited for me to fill in the words she could not express. Creating the space for her to connect with the sadness she had avoided for so long, I played the piano and sang 'Mommy, I miss you.' Repeatedly playing two chords (E, A) omitting the thirds to leave out the emotional effect of minor or major chord, I created a holding, open space. In a slow tempo, at a low register on the piano, with a subtle increase and decrease of dynamics, I invited her feelings to surface while I sang the minor third with its quality of sadness. The minor third has a quality of melancholy but also of comfort and holding as in a lullaby. My voice engaged her to emotionally go to the place she avoided, while I empathically anticipated her feelings. This plaintive mood continued through a constant centric melodic line, altered only through the changing of the chord from E to A and back. I gradually introduced the seventh interval which created more tension and seemed to pull away for a moment from the 'home' E, expressing the feeling of 'longing, but returning soon.' The repeated rhythm kept us moving forward, emotionally we walked together through the beat.

I stayed in close contact with Shelly's reactions, watching her facial expression and her body posture, careful not to overwhelm her. She smiled brightly when she heard my singing and nodded her head approvingly. For 20 minutes I sang this simple repetitive (not happy as she had requested) pattern of two chords. Similar to Diane Austin's 'holding technique'[20] I sang and included some of the following words she had told me in previous sessions:

> Mommy, I miss you so much,
> I write about you, I think about you,
> I dream about you, I play the guitar for you.
> Mommy I miss you so much,
> But I know that you can hear me.
> Can you hear me Mommy?
> I miss you so much.

Over and over again I continued the same pattern, repeating those words precisely or just keeping the basic of singing "Mommy I miss you so much." During the following weeks I repeatedly offered those sounds to her while we were building up our grieving ritual together. Over time, talking, singing and experimenting with the guitar and its soft beautiful sounds, Shelly slowly got closer to her feelings of grief. The resonance and vibration of the sounds gradually built up a releasing effect. Sometimes she sat bent over the guitar, touching some strings, and sometimes only listening to my singing and musical support. I believe we entered a deeper level of emotional connectedness, a shared trance. Through the repetition of those two chords combined with my

20. Diane Austin developed a "holding technique" of two chords to establish a predictable, secure container.

simple singing the same words, like a trance-ritual week after week, we developed a shared emotional place. As in a trance, when one is the subject of total physical, emotional and spiritual experience, I musically carried us in those frequencies of perception. While resonating together in this sound Shelly felt safe and secure enough to reach an emotional breakthrough. Sitting on the floor while my singing surrounded her, she stopped playing guitar, hid her face and finally cried; her level of existence had just expanded. I touched her back and sat with her while she crawled in my lap like a baby. I rocked, sang and comforted her. While holding her in my arms, I sang to her as a mother sings a lullaby to a child.

I believe we had entered a meditative state together and Shelly became able to cross the boundaries of her/our reality. Through carefully using my natural voice and its vibrato, possibly our nerves got attuned and affected as when singer and listener both can feel 'high' (Chapter VI). Perhaps our subconscious states were intensified while our brains were triggered, as in conditions of deep meditation and creative moments, and we experienced a state of trance. In this subconscious state, entering different worlds was easy and we were united in this moment, attuned to each other's emotional and spiritual space.

In a later moment of that important session she looked at me and with tears in her eyes asked if I am sometimes sad about death. "Yes," I said, comforting her, "and crying is okay when we are sad." She told me that crying did not help, but she seemed to feel freer after this outburst of sadness. It was the first time in three years she had shared her tears. I believe that Shelly and I shared spiritual moments as well as deeply emotional ones while creating this intimacy. To reach empathic resonance with our clients requires sensitive listening. By noticing that each speaks to us with a different voice we finally joined in "a harmonious chorus that quietly calls us home" (Wilber). Was our music therapy "home," a universal place of emotional sharing and musical understanding?

During the next session we made an audiotape of the Mommy song I had improvised so she could listen to it if she felt sad. Shelly asked me what would happen if she cried again. I assured her that it would be okay. She asked me to sing for her while she played the piano. Since we worked on her 'Mommy song' she always changed the button on piano into 'organ' or 'choir' sounds, creating a church-like or ethereal, spacey or even a bit frightening atmosphere. We created a long improvisation in the same mood as the week before. While I was repeatedly singing the same words, Shelly often looked at me and gleamed from inside. It seemed clear that my singing mirrored her thoughts and feelings and my anticipation became her expanded reality.

After this session I watched her grow emotionally, being able to face the sadness and to process the pain of the loss. She still avoided singing, but wanted to listen to our recording of the song. To prevent any emotional overload in the following session we listened to the audiotape and I videotaped her facial expressions, as I had done frequently. Whenever she heard the word 'Mommy' on the tape, she had that same gleam/glimmer/shine in her face and looked at me. I knew we were profoundly connected.

Later she was eager to watch herself carefully on the video. I had never experienced her being interested in looking at herself before. Asking me to videotape her again, she wanted to see herself smiling and playing the piano, and I understood that she was starting to like herself. Emotionally sincere, she asked for this song for her graduation ceremony at the end of the school year. I thought that it might be too personal for her and could overwhelm her. I also did not want a public performance of her inner ritual of grief, which had progressed in the safe place of individual therapy. But we were processing her feelings for the next months and found different forms for pain and happiness, including the absence of her brother, grandmother and family, or just expressing pleasure of making music together. During the Mommy song, Shelly would grow sad but slowly she sang softly with me, and later she took my hand while I sang the words she had told me about her mother. Putting her head on my lap, she started talking to her mommy while I was still singing. She was comfortable communicating with her and told me that she was sure that her mommy had heard her. Watching her doing this, I became curious if her childish fantasy had been activated or did she really reach into another level of experience? We had established a grieving singing ritual that had removed her old depressed blockage. Did we also get in touch with the lower worldspace–death?

In the following sessions Shelly was at ease with me; she gave me hugs, put her head into my lap and she shared her lovely, charming girl side with me. She decided to make a new, happy song for her mother and one for her brother. Still unsure what to express, I suggested she use some words from the book she had written. Singing about her mother and brother, we improvised two new songs: the Brother song came out in an upbeat mood, making her happy while she sang it. While practicing the songs and generally becoming more content with herself, she dared to sing them together with me in front of the video camera.

Weeks later she was equipped and emotionally prepared for the real 'happy song' about her mother, as she said, a song she would sing on the stage at the graduation performance. We made that song while improvising melodies, exchanging words and ideas very quickly. The words I offered were about the girl I saw, and she loved or rejected them without hesitation. The quality of this song was totally different from the old one: we left the monotonous grieving ritual behind us and used a lyrically up-and-down-moving melody, accompanied by changing chords. Shelly had worked through parts of the pain and had become strong and self-assured enough to express more about herself.

Removing her emotional block freed her; her body was stimulated to follow the natural flow of energy, and her body's internal system was activated. The work she accomplished to become emotionally supple and creative was ultimately a form of healing, which gave her the strength to sing the song alone. Later she even stopped my singing when I vocally supported her. Shelly was prepared to present her grief in a transformed and safe manner. I was reassured that she would not have an emotional breakdown on the stage. And in our last session before her performance, Shelly was mature enough to sing the new Mommy song comfortably by herself. During the performance, teacher and parents wept when Shelly, a bit nervous but fulfilled, sang her song:

Hi Mommy, can you hear me?
Hi Mommy, can you hear me?
I'll sing a song for you,
Can you hear my voice is singing:
Can you hear, can you hear?

Hi Mommy, can you feel me?
Hi Mommy, can you feel me?
I'll sing a song for you,
Can you feel my voice is singing:
I love you, I love you.

Hi Mommy, can you see me?
Hi Mommy, can you see me?
I became a beautiful girl,
Can you see me how I am growing:
Can you see, can you see?

Hi Mommy, can you hear me?
Hi Mommy, can you hear me?
I'll play this song for you,
Can you hear me playing the piano:
Can you hear, can you hear...?

We made this new song to honor the death of Shelly's mother, one year earlier. It helped Shelly to emotionally process the pain, to lament and understand the loss of her biological mother. Shelly's teacher observed a big improvement in the classroom and in her personal and social expression. Shelly became more conscious about herself and others' feelings, able to relate better to others by having explored her own emotions. She saw Shelly's writing skills particularly improving. Her interests and curiosity also increased; she asked more questions in the classroom and became 'alive.' Shelly still has episodes of irritability, particularly normal for her age and history, but she changed from a moody, depressed girl to a charming, awake person with more hope about her future and awareness of the world around her.

Chapter VI

In this chapter I investigate neurological brain functioning during musical vocal activities and the effect of the vibration of the voice. In *Neurological Voices* I follow Dorita Berger's explanation of old and new parts of the brain, their functions and capacities related to music. The neural network responds to musical-emotional impacts, whereby music as therapy has powerful tools to help influence chemical transformations in the body. In *Vibrating Voices* I explain that vibrato is an important natural phenomenon that can extend from the singer to listener–that both can share the same musical experience. Annette Cramer's focus on vibration of vocal sounds and importance of balanced high and low frequencies opens a different view to brain functioning in Western culture. In *Soothing Voices* I relate how Dagmar Gustorff treats coma patients, and how they respond to her soft, soothing singing, signalling their awareness of life 'outside' of the confusing experience of the coma. In *The Silent Voice* I describe a pilot study in rehabilitation in which I sang to an aphasic paralysed man and he silently communicated with me.

NEUROLOGICAL VOICES

In my work with special education, rehabilitation or psychiatric populations, I emphasize the significance of singing because it is so essential to the neurological effect or progress of clients. Singing directly affects the brain through its vibrations and I look at those aspects and its neurological function through structured vocalizations.

Singing and making up songs about feelings and ideas are especially effective tools in addressing verbal and emotional handicaps or delays, as in Shelly's case. Personal vocal expression or imitation of sound addresses speech development through the combination of rhythm, melodic line and lyrics, as follows in the case of John. A song has the ability to structure time by establishing a rhythm. Through rhythm the impulses of a person can be organized in an early stage of expression. The melody organizes the patterns of high or low tones and flows with mood changes of the person. Space for emotional expression can hereby be created and developed. The person can experience emotional satisfaction when expressing pleasure or sadness through a melody. Lyrics give meaning to the song and stimulate cognitive processes of concentration, memorization and symbolic play. Lyrics put to melody can increase the detachment of self-identification of the singer and open him or her to universal rather than only personal experience. This self-distancing effect makes it safe to 'say' something without the need for justification. These musical elements can create a container in which one can feel a sense of safety that is conducive to exploration, learning, development or relaxation, as I will describe in the rehabilitation case of Marc.

Searching for physiological explanations of this vocal impact, I wanted to look at the brain as the sensory center. I was interested to find out how clients in critical, nonverbal or comatose situations receive sound and how this vibration is neurologically perceived. Various music therapy approaches are searching for explanations about what exactly is happening in our brains during music. Still, there is no clear answer on how music is processed. Dorita Berger (2002) in her book, *Music Therapy, Sensory Integration and the Autistic Child,* presents the two-way processing of information as follows:

- input enters and goes to the brain via sensory neurons
- output comes from the brain to the body via motor neurons.

Humans have some 12 billion neurons and a constant stream of electrical impulses flows through sensory receptors along the spinal cord up to the brain. The spinal cord, brain stem, reticular activating system, amygdala, thalamus, hypothalamus, hippocampus, cerebellum and other parts, and the cerebral hemispheres register and decode this sensory input. Every major sensory system is actually being stimulated simultaneously all the time, non-stop! The human system is bombarded with millions of sensations, which the brain has either to ignore, organize or process to finally feel safe, comfortable or activated. During sensory processing humans as well as animals react to the environment first emotionally, responding from the intuitive, emotional instincts of survival. Thinking and analysing, acting from a logical level, comes later. The cortical, cognitive brain functioning needs to wait for the sub-cortical level of fear and comfort to settle down before it can work (Berger).

From different neurological sources I have learned that the human brain can be divided into two brains: the emotional, sub-cortical brain, and the cognitive, neo-cortical brain. The emotional brain is older than the cognitive brain from an evolutionary standpoint, some 500 million years old. It is the part of the brain we inherit from our animal ancestors. Within this brain there is a very thick bundle of nerves, called the 'reticular activating system.' Here, incoming information is continually sifted for discarding or distributing to other regions of the brain[21]. Sensory information is received in the limbic system's amygdala, thalamus, hypothalamus and allied regions, where assessment is made regarding safety or danger. If the information is deemed to be dangerous,

21. 75% of incoming sensory information is not needed.

the fear or fight/flight response goes into effect, calling upon the thyroid, adrenal glands and emergency units to trigger sweating, hyperventilation, increased heart rate, and similar responses, without any cognitive input to this process. When and if this information is sent further, it is logged into memory by the hippocampus, a part of the limbic system, which sequences and tags incoming stimuli for future recall. However, some traumatic experiences may reach the hippocampus, and forever be stored in the memory of the amygdala, never reaching cognition (Berger).

The intense effects of fear or pleasure may stay in long-term memory for a lifetime. Persons who may have suffered unpleasant experiences in the early years of life may have those memories stored as 'trauma' within the amygdala. During a lifetime a human will always react from this memory, where the earliest moments of protection and survival are saved. For traumatized individuals, little triggers from the environment can suddenly stir up and reactivate existential fears and feelings of discomfort, and fight/flight responses. In the case of autistic patterns, but also during coma and serious psychotic states, the sensory system is continually overstimulated: it receives information which cannot be easily decoded and compensates by shutting down. To change the old memory and build new levels of comfort and well-being, therapy treatments, especially those with music, can stimulate recoding of negative experiences and create new, more comfortable response alternatives (Berger).

The counterpart of the emotional brain is the cognitive brain, home of language, thinking and analysis of the environment. This neo-cortical (neo = new in Greek) part of the brain was developed only some 5 million years ago. It is the center of awareness and reflection where we create and work out our sense of reality. Both the sub- and neo-cortical parts of the brains are able to work separately and influence our lives. When they are connecting emotional and cognitive experiences harmonically, we are in a balanced state, also called 'flow.' If both parts of the brain are split for a long time, the possibility of illness increases. Both cortical networks include all life experiences and connect them to a form of 'emotional intelligence' as Goleman calls it in his bestseller, using our human neurological capacities (Bossinger, 2005).

The cognitive brain helps us separate, reflect and control issues that are threatening or comforting. This neo-cortical part is separated into two hemispheres, which communicate constantly with each other and each of which has its own responsibilities. The right hemisphere controls left side of the body; the left hemisphere controls the right side of the body. The right hemisphere is thought to be the instinctive and intuitive side of perception and behaviour, holistic processing of information; here is where music, creativity and speech prosody are processed. The left brain is detail-oriented, analysing facts, figures, and understanding language grammar (Berger). New forms of science assume that when both sides are resonating in the same rhythm and becoming attuned to each other, for example through breathing, humming or singing, humans are able to reach states of ecstasy, meditation and trance. During these states the neurological network is synchronized through increased alpha, theta and delta waves in the brain, creating individual as well as collective experiences of transcendence (Bossinger).

Human behaviour derives first from emotion, and afterwards from thought. Although each person may react differently, s/he follows the same pattern: first something relaxes or activates the body and later one thinks about what it was. If fear, stress and discomfort preoccupy life, the individual cannot relax and less information can reach the cognitive brain (neo-cortex). Negative memory needs time to adjust to new experiences of calmness and to remove its old information before higher learning can happen. First the sub-cortical level of fear needs attention before anything else can happen. Therefore the first important goal of therapy is creating a stress-free, non-threatening comfort level to attain a sense of calmness[22]. This is perhaps most readily achievable through music.

Music has the power to calm down the nervous system and to help create a sense of comfort. The brain's chemical reaction to emotions can be changed by music[23]. Sound reaches into old part of the brain, activates the sub-cortical, emotional network, which can create chemical changes. The neuronal network responds to the musical-emotional impact through its chemical transformation. Intensive repetition of musical or vocal therapy interventions may reinforce a sense of safety and the chemical change activates new neuronal learning. Specifically applied, music can touch the limbic system[24], which is able to adjust the physiological system of the body and process learning.

> Music does not particularly require neo-cortex processing. Language absolutely does. Music proceeds directly through the limbic system (amygdala, thalamus, hypothalamus, hippocampus, cerebellum etc.), needing no further explanation from cortical lobes. Of course, the neo-cortex can play a convenient role in interpreting music, but this is not a

---

22. See also information about the 'triune brain' model which differentiates the brain into three parts: http://en.wikipedia.org/wiki/Triune_brain; http://www.thebrain.mcgill.ca/flash/d/d_05/d
23. Reducing the flow of cortisol and inducing the flow of dopamine [neurotransmitters], Berger, p.135. The physical system of reward and emotion in the human body reacts to music as to sex, food or drugs, even if we do not need music for survival as we do the other elements (induced dopamine).
24. Research at universities in Germany and the USA showed that regularly focused singing increased the function of the immune system. In different studies of singers in choirs, an increase of immune globulin A level was measured. In one study the intensity of the singing experience was responsible for the amount of increase. During a rehearsal the level increased 150%, during a performance 240%, dependent on the stage of pleasure and emotional involvement (Bossinger, p.127).

> requirement. Configuration of sounds will be responded to with or without "intellectual" processing. An infant understands music expression at the intuitive, sub-cortical level, without as yet having any developed "intellect" (Berger, p. 130).

Music enters through the senses and can enable humans to relax, enjoy and open their system without interpretations and fear. The neo-cortical processing is not necessary but it can help in the later development of emotions and intellect through understanding and correcting behaviour. Music creates a sense of safety and security where emotional and cognitive processes–for example feelings and language skills–are facilitated through sensory integration. The voice can especially instill inflections and prosody in persons with autism, many of whom tend toward monotonal speech (Berger).

John was a 9-year-old nonverbal autistic boy whose speech development was enabled through sound in the form of structured rhythm, tone, melody and my attuned personal vocal expression. Besides speech and language, John was developing emotional and cognitive skills during our music therapy work. Through his strong love for music and imitation of my singing sounds, he learned to relax and to feel comfortable in a musical environment. From there he picked up sounds and learned words or song lyrics and he understood their meaning. The teacher in the classroom noticed his new verbalizations when he started to sing words of the songs he had heard in music therapy. She intensified his daily speech practice and I worked twice a week with him concentrating on singing words and phrases. The song lyrics, production of nonsense vocal sounds, and imitation of my sounds organized John's language articulation. Stimulating his exhalation of tones, his brain could learn 'how to exhale sounds,' relax him and later shape sounds into letter sounds and words (Berger, p. 144). It seemed that in his case all brain functions were cooperating and an opening for his higher cognitive processing became possible.

John's progress was rapid; after 6 months of intensive therapy, he could recognize and point to the objects of the words he was pronouncing. His newly developed skills will help him to improve himself in the world of speech and to express and communicate his needs and desires. His progress was possible through vocal music therapy strategies using tone, melody, rhythm, and lyrics to stimulate the brain in many areas simultaneously.

This multisensory integration process through music and voice has important value also in neurology and rehabilitation for speech development or recovery by aphasia, stroke and Alzheimer's patients, and improved movement by Parkinson's sufferers[25].

---

25. See Aldridge (2005), Music Therapy and Neurological Rehabilitation.

VIBRATING VOICES

Another music therapist, Annette Cramer, offers some facts about the neurological effects of vocal frequencies and vibrations on the brain. A musician, philosopher, psychologist and music therapist from Germany, Cramer combines neurological knowledge and traditional approaches to the voice in her work and in her innovative book about the voice (1998, *Das Buch von der Stimme*). She describes in detail the vibrato of the voice and the frequencies of the vibration in the body as important concepts for intense attention. She supposes that the tendency in our Western societies to prefer lower female and male voices and filter out the high frequencies of the voice is not healthy behaviour. This filtering, evident in many sound recordings, movies and discotheques, is an attempt to placate us with low sounds–whether we want them or not! (See also Chapter IV.)

Our ears need high frequencies to stimulate normal brain functioning. The main area of hair cells in the ear reacts to high tones and less to low ones. On activation of the hair cells, impulses go to the cerebral cortex and transport vital energy in the form of stimuli. These stimuli arouse the capacity for concentration, the balance in the body and the sensorial movement.

Referencing the research of Rohmert (1994) about the trained voices of singers, Cramer describes the intense neurological relationship between a singer and a listener (p. 210). The high frequencies in the voice of a singer create significant neurological signals: they vibrate and stimulate the hair cells in the ear of singer and listener, which activates their formatio reticularis: the concentration, attention or awake-center of the brain and the connected brain functions. The formatio reticularis is activated continuously through the voice because of the stimuli connection of the nerves in the ear to this nerve network. Such connected brain functions include the limbic system, which is responsible for emotions and for primitive drives and instincts–the older part of the brain, as described above.

It is possible to activate the nerve networks of both singer and listener through the three frequencies of 3000, 5000 and 8000 Hz. The reason for this–besides the activation of the hair cells–are the high frequency signals of the formatio reticularis itself: in the same frequency ranges (3000, 5000 and 8000 Hz), this nerve network sends signals and activates the brain–thereby creating resonance[26] with itself. In deep states of meditation, these signals are audible as 'inner tones.' Through singing tones with the same high frequencies, brain training can be achieved, keeping or intensifying its cells in self-resonance. This

26. Resonance is a physical phenomenon where two systems come into vibrational alignment or similarity.

brain activation is possible through the trained voice of a singer, but Cramer is convinced that an untrained voice can also reach some of these parameters with the similar or same effect. The listener and performer of high vocal sound can share the same sensations as feeling 'high,' (a light form of trance), feeling awake, or increased concentration or sensitivity. Low tone frequencies resonate in the ear with larger amplitude and can be felt deep in the entrails. The lower sound is easier to perceive in the body and helps to ground people and can also elicit trance conditions. Both high and low frequencies are needed for a balanced and healthy brain functioning. Therefore regularly singing, with a trained or untrained voice, together or alone, supports the neurological and emotional balance of health.

Besides frequency, other physical phenomena of the singer can be transferred to listener, if the latter is open for it. For example, slow or fast breath can relax or activate; the frequencies of vibrato can regulate body functions and stimulate speech expression. The vibrato of a voice has an important role on the brain and body sensations. Cramer explains that vibrato is not only a technical but also a natural phenomenon, that appears when the body is totally integrated in the vocal sound. The vibrato is a rhythmical swaying of the pitch of the tone, which is connected to the simultaneous swaying of the volume and timbre. The swaying must fall within a certain amplitude and frequency so the tones hold a pleasant suppleness, tenderness and richness. A vibrato between 4 and 7 Hz is common for a singer's voice and can trigger the brain to vibrate with the same frequency, resulting in the Theta condition of between 4 and 7 Hz. These frequencies are the same as in conditions of creative moments and deep meditation. Also the heart and blood pressure system can be regulated through the vibrato because the waves of blood circulation sway in the same vibration of 7 Hz in the human skeleton (Bentov in Cramer). Furthermore, communicative expression gets inspired through vibrato because the speech center in the brain resonates at 6 Hz[27].

Using our voices causes our brain to respond. Talking and singing activate cortical centers; talking more the left side, and singing more the right side, as discussed above. The neurological impact of singing has profound effects because of its deep penetration into sub-cortical levels, while talking effects mostly neo-cortical levels. Although I have listened to every possible human utterance in order to understand its ability to help us find personal and collective harmony, I realize that there is so much more to learn about the results of vocal vibration in order to use it effectively in therapy. The benefit of repeated daily singing as 'medicine' during the times of middle age and in various cultures, mirrors ancient knowledge of vocal therapy. Singing has

---

27. See also Robert Jourdain about the connection between music and the brain.

helped treat physical and psychological diseases for centuries; now we need the scientific knowledge to research, restore, and repropagate these olds forms.

SOOTHING VOICES

One ancient form of vocal treatment is the soothing lullaby and its related vocal sounds. In the section about the acoustic symbols in Chapter III, I explained how the babbling sound of an infant is repetitive and relaxes the baby and, most of the time, also the mother. The mother learns how to distinguish the relaxed from the pained sound of her baby, and when she sings, she uses the same simple repetitive sound patterns. Her voice–untrained, smooth or rough–will be the most effective in soothing, relaxing and comforting her infant, perhaps because of the intense vibrational, neurological and emotional connection between mother and child. It is vital to learn that an adult in pain, like a baby, is hungering for the same comfort. It's important to keep in mind that many adults were as infants comforted by a female singing voice. In crisis situations, such as accidents, illnesses and times of deep sorrow, we often regress and desire to be hugged and treated as a baby or a child. Also during extremely serious conditions such as comatose states, adults wish somebody would softly sing to them, to feel that there is human life 'outside' of the coma.

Dr. Dagmar Gustorff (2000) is a German music therapist who works in an intensive care unit with comatose patients. She found that in a comatose condition, the patient is sensitive to human connection and that the quality of such connection can sometimes determine whether a patient lives or dies. People in coma often live in a prolonged quasi-psychotic state of consciousness. Like a dream where nothing is clear, everything is flexible and changeable. During coma the skill to organize impressions and experiences is missing. Reality is mixed with dreamy contexts and illusions, and patients are living in a world of fantasy. In such a state of mind, one patient organized his experience of staff members through connecting to their voices: for every voice and name he imagined a body and head fitting onto it. But sometimes his organizational skill became confused and he would have bodies without heads or heads without a fitting body.

Many patients describe feeling 'imprisoned' and losing their autonomy during a comatose condition. Others experience their condition as being in war, accident, illness or death. Doctors and nurses are misperceived as 'criminals,' 'prison wardens,' and 'slaveholders' (patient's experiences in Gustorff, p. 132). The staff should be extremely alert to comatose patients' potential for fearful and disorientated perceptions. It seems that the analytical skill for a reality check is not working and the patient experiences the environment mainly through emotional levels. The comatose patient might need a 'mirroring' of his perception, similar to the tender contact between mother and child, to build up rapport. The noisy intensive care unit and the loud commands of staff, such as 'Open your eyes!' undermine the patient's need for softness and personal contact. One patient awoke from a comatose condition saying that he had not wanted to 'come back to life' at one point because of the harsh sounds around him.

Gustorff found that many coma patients responded positively when sung to. Through her voice, Gustorff carefully attuned to the patient's condition, searching for the entrance to a common world-space. Patients reported having extremely vivid and interesting experiences when receiving sensitive vocal treatment. One of her patients explained that the singing was a wonderful, 'more than beautiful,' intense experience when the music therapist was connecting with her heart and staying there. Through the singing, she was able to come out from the darkness through a tunnel and into the brightness. These amazing experiences of coma patients teach us to understand the serious and significant role of singing empathically.

Singing and resonating with another, being empathically connected– these are the moments where we can share the different levels of experience with each other. Singing without words with the natural vibrato of her voice was the only contact that reached one of Gustorff's clients to call her back to life:

> The music was exquisite. The first time I didn't recognize it as a voice, but as some kind of medieval wind instrument. But the second time I knew it was a voice, that there was a person there, there was someone who didn't want to kill me (Gustorff in Ansdell, p. 59).

This patient is well now and lives a normal life. He is still thankful for Dr. Gustorff's help; the subtle vocal music gave him his life back.

The vocal sounds she was using matched her client's breathing rhythm:

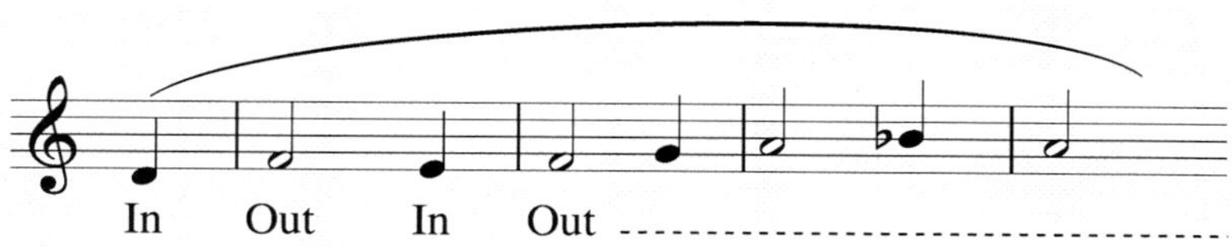

The comfort of her soothing and relaxing voice reached his consciousness. The simple, primitive melody Gustorff used provided the acoustic symbols as a synchronic natural answer to his need for this purely personal experience. As demonstrated, it is possible to comfort adults through vocal music therapy in medical settings. Using the voice in this way is recommended for the first moments of contact with extremely weak or disoriented patients, because it reaches into universal human memory of the emotional (old) brain, connecting to primal moments of security, the most direct relationship from 'I' to 'you' (Baumann in Gustorff). And being unconscious, as in coma, does not mean being without perception or the need for sensitive treatment. Through the sensitive use of the voice, we can awaken our storehouse of natural forms of cure and care that we still carry within us. Through entrainment[28], we can vocally and energetically contact and pull people into rhythmic and harmonic resonance, with and even without their notice.

Simply, easily and inexpensively, we can comfort our patient's fears and howls through our own use of vocal human sounds. With familiarity and understanding of the patient's background, using their and our acoustic symbols, our voices can heal. In multicultural societies, in concentrated places like hospitals, institutions, medical and psychiatric clinics, schools and community centers, where different mentalities, cultures, languages and behaviours merge, the need for every kind of increased understanding is indisputable.

THE SILENT VOICE – A CASE EXAMPLE

For a pilot study I have conducted in a rehabilitation setting, I worked with patients who were strongly isolated, physically handicapped, and emotionally and cognitively confused; most were without speech. These patients received no other form of treatment other than what was required for their basic needs. During the study I measured my client's blood pressure every session directly before and after my vocal treatment. My singing voice effected changes in the most of the sessions: blood pressure would decrease when my vocal treatment approach was soothing; when my approach was more stimulating, often there was a rise in blood pressure. This significant impact encouraged me to focus more attention on the correlation between singing and therapy, especially in the area of relaxation. Focusing on the affective, relational, cognitive and physical levels of a given situation, my approach often shifted while singing, as I will illustrate in the following example with a nonverbal client. Using my analytical categorization of different aspects of the voice (see Chapter VII), being alert to his levels I was able to effect a transformation of them.

---

28. The scientific theory of entrainment suggests that the order and coherence of certain kinds of music can energetically pull an unbalanced individual into rhythmic and harmonic resonance with it. Musical entrainment is a passive yet powerful phenomenon that often occurs without conscious awareness (Montello, p. 39).

Marc is 90-year-old African American male who had a cerebro-vascular accident many years ago and was totally dependent on nursing care. He had gastro-intestinal bleeding, a urinary tract infection, and was paralysed on the left side of his body. He was dysphasic, lethargic, and limited in orientation and responses. He was nearly always lying in bed except for short periods sitting in a wheelchair. Marc was not able to initiate any verbal contact, and did not interact with anybody in the hospital other than what was necessary during daily nursing procedures.

The affective level of my approach was emotional, soft, and calming because of Marc's serious medical conditions. With a whispering, smooth or soft voice–in sharp contrast to the nurses and doctors with their loud vocal sounds–I tried to develop intimacy and a trusting contact. Connecting myself to his rhythm of breath I carefully sang a greeting improvisation. I believe, as I described with the comatose states, human beings in these serious conditions become disoriented and fearful and hunger for comfort the way babies do. Sometimes when I sang to him, I found myself feeling like a mother singing to a baby. Marc seemed helpless, abandoned and unprotected to me and this brought up my own feelings of countertransference as a mother needing to comfort her child. Through my therapeutic presence and understanding, I vocally became aware of and then worked with my countertransference to meet his needs. Marc was unable to verbally express his needs. I assumed he needed a form of shared friendly human contact. Once in a while his daughter came to visit him. She told me that her father understood language and that he could hear sounds. She also told me that he loved music, especially old traditional American and Gospel songs. And so I adjusted my approach accordingly.

My level of relational interaction acted as a subtle developmental intervention with Marc. Having begun by relaxing him through singing as mother to baby, now I also stimulated Marc and brought the outside adult world into his room by singing familiar songs for him. The shifts in the relational communication pattern were delicate and it was important for me to stay focused on his need and not on my own feelings of counter-transference. He wasn't only as he appeared; he was an old man with life experiences and both the baby and the adult needed care, attention and contact. Singing songs of his past, I tried to connect him to his memory and emotion of times he was well. Mindful of what his daughter told me, I often sang "Oh, What a Wonderful World," "Amazing Grace" or other songs familiar to him. Once when I was softly humming the melody of Amazing Grace he reacted with slow movements of his left paralysed arm and leg when previously only the right side of his body had shown movement.

I approached him on the cognitive level through his background and present life condition. My intention was to break for a short moment the isolation between Marc and the world. I wanted to give him an opportunity to truly feel human contact and communication. I sang and improvised songs, hummed and once in a while talked to him. I started every session with a 'Hello' or 'Good Morning' improvisation, using the symbolic language of vocal sounds, short poems or parts of songs as text. The contents were images of nature, the weather, and what I had noticed about him–the usual things of the day. The Good-Bye's included information about when I would return. Because of his isolated life, I believed that he needed pure human contact as well as clear communication about daily orientation, information about my presence, schedules and purpose of my visits. I sang only songs familiar to him, even though he could not sing or respond, so that he might enjoy memories around these songs. I did not use any new song with a high, unknown or intellectual level of content, because of his current, limited condition.

My aesthetic approach accepted any natural sound or movements he made, and I learned to respect them. This was not always easy for me because of his offensive smell and his authentic, unusual, limited sounds and behaviour, like sighing, yawning, and falling asleep. My voice imitated, adapted or commented on his sounds and finally moved into sound as pure human contact–a form of transparency[29]. I also interacted with him using peaceful, light vocal sounds to acknowledge the need for human sound in his room. His responses to my music were minimal: his eyes were active and searched for orientation and contact–maybe for the source of the sound he heard. His body made tiny, slow arm and leg movements, and his breathing was irregular and erratic with gasps and sighs. He yawned and swallowed very often, which could possibly have been an emotional response to his stimulated body and mind. His breathing sounded like a death rattle and I often interacted with these sounds through relaxed breathing in the same rhythm and later through vocally comforting him. It seemed he relaxed when I sang because his blood pressure went down[30]. He made sounds like 'Ah' and 'Oh,' just expressing his most primary feelings or possibly trying to imitate my sounds, but not in any predictable pattern.

My spiritual approach was to meet any state of consciousness he seemed to present. Even when he did not react at all to the music and he seemed to be sleeping, I continued singing. I often repeated my melodies until I became a part of the sound myself and transcended it. I found that a simple centric melody or the repetition of only two tones were often effective in creating little ritualistic forms just as in ancient healing rituals. I tried to become totally

29. Transparence: quality of state of being transparent; passing through different states and qualities of sounds to finally become sound. Transcendence: quality of state of being transcendent; going beyond ordinary limits; surpassing; exceeding.

30. I measured M's blood pressure before and after our session. I put the pulse collar on his right, non-paralyzed arm between his elbow and wrist and did not move it until the end of the session. This way I could guarantee that the measurement would take place at the same point throughout the session.

present through my own simple sound and my connection to him. I moved from actively making sound into being the sound by tuning myself into feelings in the surrounding environment. Using my shamanistic as well as vocal training and experiences I knew that my/our reality could expand into his whole room. I felt that I created a space through my own vibration and included Marc in this sensation. I hoped that I could connect him to something bigger than himself.

Technically speaking, I sang softly in simple patterns and often used descending minor second and third intervals, rising fourths, fifths and sixths, and half tones for variations between the intervals and microtones. I used these intervals intuitively and analysed them later. During a single session I usually sang in the same key for improvisations and songs so as to simplify the musical material used. Sensitive to his appearance and cultural background, I improvised melodies in lullaby, blues, gospel or spiritual style in simple repeating patterns. Later in a session, I would add familiar songs. These I sang with fuller voice to stimulate him more. I experimented with my vibrato in the moment and changed it when I felt the sound needed to become smaller or more intimate. I then repeated the melodies of the familiar songs with improvisations of words to finish the session, as described above.

Throughout a session I was aware of the difference between a performing voice and Marc's need for intimate sounds. I sang the improvisations more softly and with personal intention in order better be able to respond to his needs. Often I tried to sing in the rhythm of his breathing or to catch his pattern to make a direct connection to him. But he would continue the rhythm I was making only for a short while and then he would hold his breath as though he were concentrating. Sometimes I sang in my rhythm and after a while M. would adapt his breathing rhythm to my singing, seemingly in response to my singing. But all of his patterns and reactions were inconsistent, so it is impossible to draw any conclusions. However, my physical voice experiences allowed me to observe his body patterns. Even when his cognitive capacities seemed limited, I believe that the music gently penetrated his isolation and accessed his inner world. My experience and awareness of my own physical conditions helped me understand how to perceive vocal vibration and how to direct it towards Marc and into the room. The resonance and effect of my sound was intensely dependent on the level of relaxation or tension in my own body as well as his. I believe this vibrational contact connected Marc with himself, his brain, his body, and with me, his environment.

Because of Marc's nonverbal and limited condition the measurements I relied on were my observations during the sessions, analysis of videotapes and the changes in his blood pressure. In a study by Condon (Cramer), when every micromovement of the body and all the words and syllables of a conversation were analysed it was discovered that the speaker's micro movement in the communication was synchronized to the micro-units of the words they used. All movements followed the same metric time and connected every syllable, word and sentence in perfect rhythm with movements of the body. The listener's movements synchronized with the speech and movement patterns of the speaker. This communication interaction looked like a dance. The only requirement for this dance was the inner motivation and interest in the communication. If I apply this idea to Marc's responses, I understand better his reactions and possibly his blood pressure changes. During the eight sessions I had with him, his blood pressure decreased six times (with sometimes an increase in pulse) and increased two times. My approach for every session was to stimulate him in a calming, gentle way. In the six sessions when the blood pressure went down, he was stimulated in a smooth and soft way. He yawned frequently and he looked at me, maybe searching for the source of the sound. Sometimes his breathing adapted to the rhythm of the music, and in general he relaxed. Maybe we communicated with each other in some strange dance form. In session four Marc was more active than ever before and his blood pressure went up. In this session there was environmental noise, which could have created stress; I had also brought another therapist to help me with the videotaping. It seemed that M. reacted more spontaneously to everything that happened in that session. He made little sounds and he reacted more to my sounds.

Is it possible that the impact of a second person and environmental noise–big changes in daily life for a person in isolation–strongly affect authentic behavior? There were no other known influences, such as a different time of the day, medical changes or visits. Possibly we were not in the same rhythmic pattern of our conversation. In session six he was sleeping before and during the initial phase of my treatment. While I was singing to him he woke up and his blood pressure went up. Such a change in blood pressure is normal after sleeping.

My experiences with Marc have demonstrated to me the measurable physical effects of my vocal interventions. His reactions and my knowledge about the vibration of the voice led me to believe that my treatment was completely worthwhile. It connected this isolated man–even if only for moments–to the world outside of himself, to other human beings and his environment. In situations where the therapist barely gets any feedback about the needs of the client, we have to trust our own intuition even more, using the awareness and knowledge of our body as instrument and the voice as tool for navigation.

Chapter VII

This last chapter of music therapy practice involves an analysis of the clinical vocal interventions and therapeutic techniques I have developed and categorized. With *Methodical Voices* I portray my search for the primary effect in singing: making contact with myself and my environment. Singing is penetrating and these intimate human interactions comprise the vocal communication between my clients and I that are described in *Personal Voices*. Being in true contact and communication requires complete awareness of authentic Self, including reflections about personal and professional attitude as well as acceptance of mistakes and missed opportunities. In *Vocal Interventions* I describe the qualitative, quantitative and therapeutic techniques and methods I've developed over the years. Herein I explain in detail my analytical categorization of emotional, relational, cognitive, physical, aesthetic, spiritual and technical aspects of the voice. In *The Painful Voice*, a pilot study in rehabilitation, I describe and analyse those developed methods while I vocally pacify a paralyzed stroke victim.

METHODICAL VOICES

From my work as music therapist and my clinical experiences, a vocal therapy method has emerged. I often use some of the primal vocal forms of treatment to make conscious contact with my environment: singing, humming, vocalizing, weaving in meaningful words, and expressing them directly, vocally into a melodic line. I do sing what I see, hear or feel and express it spontaneously, communicating with my surroundings. I remember doing this unconsciously and naturally when I was a child. Without any musical education, we sang at home with humour when some practical catastrophes appeared: rhyming a poem about a plate that was broken or singing a silly melody when the basement of the house was flooded. As an adult I sing in difficult moments often after shocking moments of stress, anger or tension. Making up a short melodic phrase seems to lessening the strong effect of the shock or catastrophes and helps me structure and control the anxious situation.

Through my clinical work I focused on the primary effect of this coping form of singing on others. I discovered through research that this form of spontaneous vocal expression was perhaps similar to what indigenous people all over the world did when they connected themselves with their environment. In the Part B of the book I will explain more about those cultures.

Intuitively and then later consciously I developed a therapy form in which the voice becomes the center for human interaction, often based on principles of primitive and ritualistic healing. The primitive part is the purest human expression, at every moment giving voice when pain, grief, confusion or even chaos appears. The ritualistic part structures the pain and grief from the confusion, chaotic and shocking impression into a concrete form. Simple forms are created to incorporate the expression and repetition of some of the acoustic symbols, grieving or shocking words, or only a phrase of rhythmic sing-crying and deep breathing. Cyclic and more cultivated situations also become structured through the symbolic, social form of a ritual. Forms of ritualistic singing in laments, for example, are made to enable members of the family and community to tell the dead they are missed and to share this emotion with each other (see Part B). Every repetition of the lamenting song sends out the same symbolic message with a coping effect for the pain of loss, similar to Shelly's experience as I explained above.

PERSONAL VOICES

Interactions with the songs, sounds and acoustic symbols that my clients are sending out determine my professional attitude for my future work. These symbols–their messages, the qualities of sound, and my understanding of them–are communication. According to Watzlawick, an Austrian communication psychotherapist, non-communication does not exist: every human gesture, signal, movement or sound is communication and sends messages out. Even silence is communication, with the message that there is no talk or verbalization possible.

As a therapist, I have the responsibility to try to perceive and interact with any kind of communication, including silence or unusual acoustic symbols. This task requires a special awareness as well as the provision of time in order to discover the variety of symbols that are being sent out. And it calls for a developed sensitivity to determine when it is necessary to interact with them. In the past when I entered some of my therapy sessions, I was not able to hear and interact with many of the acoustic symbols of my clients and within myself. But gradually I developed sensitivity through my own process of awareness of my vocal, bodily and kinaesthetic presence. I am still working on it and I am sure that the process will never end. The more I discover about my Self, the more I realize how important this knowledge is in fostering the therapeutic relationship.

When I listen to a tape or see a video of one of my therapy sessions, I still can hear and see some missed interactions. For example, I hear my own voice talking or singing, not soft and smooth as my intention was to comfort the client, but much more tense and impatient. I thought I had been singing smoothly and comfortably, I sought to be empathic but the tape showed me that I wasn't. My vocal sounds on the tape showed at times that I was not aware of my presence. The same has occurred during observations of the work of my colleagues. Watching them during their work, I discovered we all have our blind spots and miss important moments of interaction. At times I observed an experienced therapist singing a song with a beautiful performing voice, but unable to meet the client. On the other extreme are therapists who are uncomfortable or inexperienced with their voices, singing or uttering disconnected or repulsive sounds. How often we are aware of moments like that: not daring to sing, singing for ourselves or being occupied with our personal needs and fears. At those times we are not listening presently to our body and voices and we will miss the client if we are not authentic.

As therapists, the subtle awareness of our presence through what we do and how we are in therapy is crucial for me. *Doing* is the intensely active performance of our thoughts and desires. *Being* is the integrated process of perception of the Self, including its irreducible duality of thoughts and emotions. It is the totality of the personality with internalised awareness of life experiences, our capacities and our limitations. It is the true spiritual existence which transcends and includes all.

Even after many years of work, this process needs to be continued for the development of an authentic personality, an authentic Self. Being able to be an authentic Self influences my personal and professional attitude. This authentic Self can integrate my sounds of twilight and shadow, as well as bright daylight, which exist clearly in my voice. I have written about the importance of the impact of the doctor's voice in the healing process of the client and I believe this is no different for the music therapist.

An authentic Self with awareness of its vocal presence and its effects is able to really trust the process of personal and professional growth: to accept mistakes and missed opportunities, to listen to one's own acoustic mirror and its messages, and to continuously integrate all of these aspects into the process of growth. Growth only comes through understanding of this endless process of awareness. And the voice can be the most vital tool for navigation in this process.

To use the voice for effective therapy is to practice and ground an authentic, united Self. Through spontaneous, individual, vocal expression, in ritualistic as well as therapeutic forms, bridges are being built between human beings and the environment. The voice as a tool for navigation and as an acoustic mirror of the personality is the key to human contact. In order to support and illuminate this insight and to stimulate personal growth for myself and for others, I have created the following interventions. These are my own experiences and they could be used as applications for voicework in music therapy.

VOCAL INTERVENTIONS

In my clinical work, I have used different vocal techniques for specific clients and therapy goals. Through my voice workshops with Kate Geller, we have distilled those techniques for broader use and generalized them for our voicework and clinical approaches. We have separated these techniques into qualitative, quantitative and therapeutic uses of the voice. The qualitative/quantitative techniques show examples for what to do vocally to become aware of the bodily aspects, its support and possibilities for achieving therapy goals. The therapy methods expose how vocal inventions can be used to determine levels of development. But first I will simply start with breath and voice instructions.

VOCAL TECHNIQUES. Breathing and focusing intensely on inhaling and exhaling opens the body and senses. Breathe fully and 'tune' yourself; allow more oxygen flow into your body affecting blood, skin, organs, brain and every cell of body. If you have no previous voice training, simply imagine the vocal sounds described and try them out; discover the differences in sounds and feeling. While softly vocalizing these sounds, always stay in touch with how it *feels,* not how it *sounds*. Change what you are doing if it feels uncomfortable or painful. When your voice becomes dry, husky or hoarse, rest for a while. Drink lots of fluids, water or warm tea to regulate the mucus of vocal cords. Get enough sleep; do not vocalize under stress; do not force vocal cords to vibrate with intense pressure and vocalize in a relaxed state if you are not trained. Vocalizing and singing develops only through practice not through reading voice instruction books. Some books are very helpful, look for example at Hewitt, Linklater, and Gardner-Gordon or see Part C of this book for instructions from our voice workshops. But most importantly–*sing*.

Qualitative: the following vocal techniques are for awareness and purposeful structuring of the different qualities of vocal sound:

- Centering the body–vocal activity with full body support: breathing, whispering, laughing and screaming as well as cultivated singing
- Freeing the voice: unlimited vocalizations in any position, activating some areas, relaxing others

- Being present in the moment: connecting the voice with feelings and words that emerge; becoming attuned to one's own inner resources

Quantitative: the following vocal techniques are for various kinds of vocal sounds:

- Singing in the chest or middle register, or head register for special effects
- Singing and humming softly with an airy sound
- Singing thinly and purely like wind instruments
- Singing with open or forced resonance, clear and direct sound
- Singing with and without vibrato

THERAPEUTIC VOCAL METHODS. The following table is an attempt to structure my experiences during any kind of vocal expression, and to categorize the therapeutic use of this vocal intervention on different levels:

Affective Level–human expression. Uttering primary sounds:

- sighing, babbling, laughing, crying, screaming, groaning, singing, silence
- information revealed in the quality in the voice:
  - emotions: anger, grief, fear, pleasure
  - moods: love, shock, embarrassment, jealousy

Relational Level–human contact. Communicating through the voice and body:

- calling, telling, talking, singing, silence
- soothing, nurturing, holding, comforting
- stimulating, provoking, invoking, grieving, inspiring, confronting, protecting

Cognitive Level–symbolic representation. Giving meaning through words, melodies, imagery:

- focusing on content: humming, syllables, names, phrases, poetry, compositions
- stimulating concentration and memories
- bridging the external world to the client's internal world and vice versa
- incorporating the client's symbols into a symbolic language

Physical Level–corporeal attunement. Producing body-centered vocal sound:

- vibrating the voice in and around the body
- experiencing the resonance of the voice in the body
- modulating relaxation and tension in the body
- acknowledging a neurological response to frequencies of vocal sounds

Aesthetic Level–authentic appreciation. Discovering beauty in any vocal sound:

- opening the senses and especially the ears to receive any human sound
- accepting the attraction and repulsion of human sounds
- appreciating cultural origins in natural, authentic sounds
- recognizing a transparence of the client's inner world in the sound of the voice

Spiritual Level–vocal transcendence. Experiencing levels of consciousness:

- inducing trance-like states through vocal repetition
- expanding the sense of reality, place, and time through intense, focused vocalization
- transitioning from 'doing' into 'being' through conscious breathing and sound vibration

Technical Level–vocal skills. Using the body as a musical instrument:

- producing breath and tone;
- developing accurate pitch, vibrato, overtones
- differentiating performance and intimate vocal sound
- expanding vocal range: affect, dynamic, pitch, style (including difference musical cultures)
- studying human anatomy involved in producing vocal sound: larynx, diaphragm, lungs, ribs, spine, abdominal and back musculature, etc.

THE PAINFUL VOICE – A CASE EXAMPLE

These levels of therapeutic vocal methods and techniques are so various that I want to offer more in-depth explanation. I explained in the case example in Chapter VI more about a pilot study I conducted in a rehabilitation setting. While there I studied the direct effect of the singing voice on the most traumatized patients and through these case examples, I analysed my work in detail.

The highest functioning client I worked with in this rehabilitation setting was a patient in his seventies, Paul, who suffered from a stroke, was paralyzed on the left side of his body and dependent on a wheelchair for getting around. Paul had a history of high blood pressure, was cognitively alert with a sarcastic sense of humor and slowed verbal skills. In his former life Paul was a professional with a leadership position, but since his illness he had totally lost strength, comfort and control over his life. Dependent on nursing care, he suffered emotionally and physically trying to adjust to the changes in his life, experiencing pain, discomfort and a high level of confusion. I used my voice with him in different ways, operating with a variety of vocal methods and techniques. Connecting on the **relational level** I sang a mixture of songs with diverse forms of contact. When I sang songs like "Que Será Será" or "Let It Be" to inspire, nurture or relax Paul, in difficult moments he remembered those songs and told me later that he had sung the songs to himself in frustrating situations. He used those songs while waiting in the elevator with nurses and aides who would not inform him where they were taking him. Paul was dialoguing with himself. Feelings of being "a package with no identity," he said, increased his frustration and confusion. The offered songs created a confrontation with his condition, stimulating grieving, later comforting him and finally helping him to cope. I sometimes sang to him with a provocative but responsible, clear and direct sound, or sometimes we were holding together the silence of 'being lost.'

I also often talked with Paul about his nightmares, feelings of fear and of being lost amidst his serious psychological and physical conditions. We made a clear connection between the contents of the songs we used, those he requested or ones I chose for him. Their symbolic representation and the meanings for him linked to his **cognitive level**. Sometimes I started with a vocal improvisation in response to a question or comment of his. Paul often was frustrated that everybody visiting his room had no time for him. Especially when he was in pain, he experienced nurses and doctors enter and leave the room, rushed and irritated. When I entered and established my music equipment in his room, Paul asked me surprised: "Do you have time?" I did not directly answer his question, acknowledging his confusion, but I sang back to him "Yes, I have time for you, I have time to sing for you." I made a long improvisation out of his repeated verbal and nonverbal comments. He silently looked at me and finally with a thankful facial expression, he relaxed while receiving my singing:

I Have Time For You

transcribed by Phil Stockli

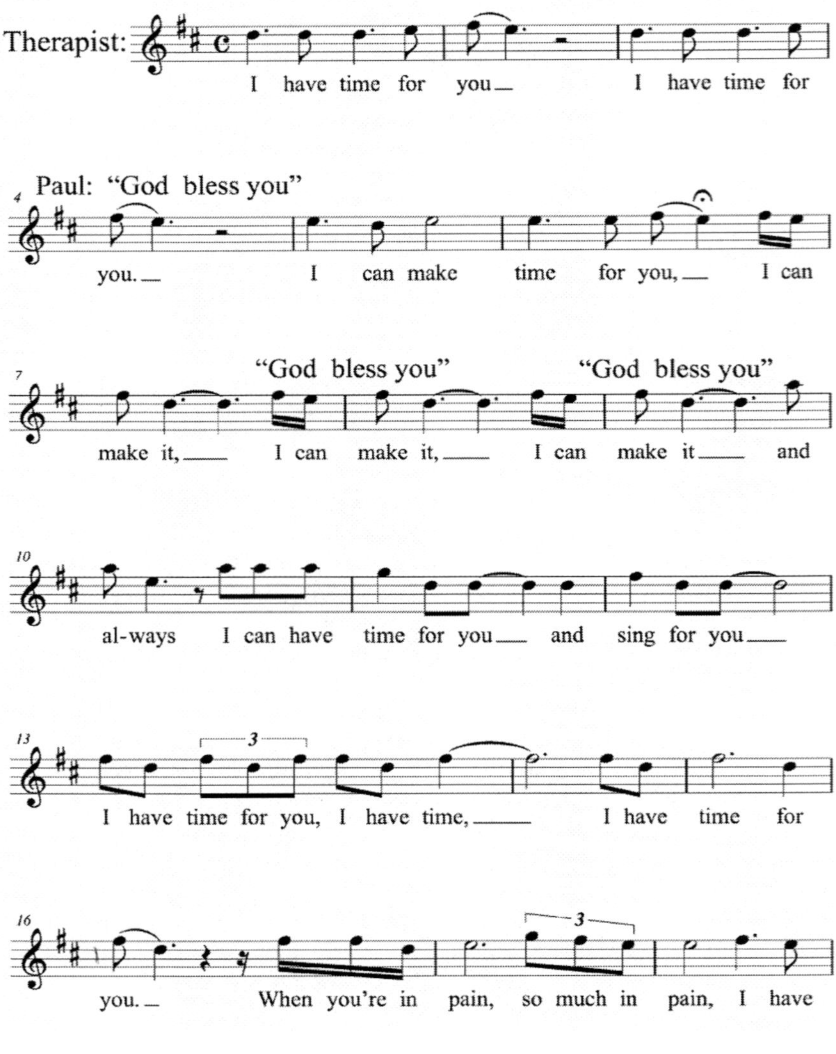
Therapist:
I have time for you I have time for
4
Paul: "God bless you"
you. I can make time for you, I can
7
"God bless you" "God bless you"
make it, I can make it, I can make it and
10
al-ways I can have time for you and sing for you
13
3
I have time for you, I have time, I have time for
16
3
you. When you're in pain, so much in pain, I have

I Have Time For You

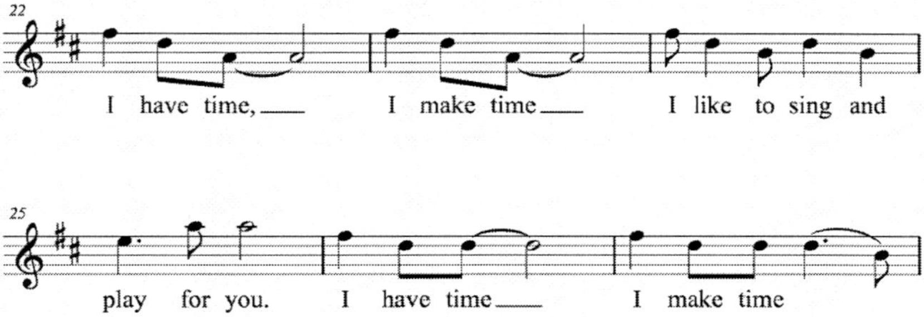
22
I have time,
I make time
I like to sing and
25
play for you.
I have time
I make time

Often I repeated or mirrored his words, integrating them into the song, and our conversations would continue this way. I picked up words Paul offered about his difficult situation, improvised them lyrically, and he responded verbally. I was able to vocally break his isolation, to hold his sarcastic, negative and humorous comments in the music and to react in an appropriate way–supportive, exaggerative, and funny–absorbing and containing him. Like call and response I incorporated his personal symbols into language or song.

I would sing Paul's name in the improvisations, connecting on the **affective level**. Through listening to my voice, the value of his own name took on a new meaning for him and he choked with emotion. Through the quality of my personal voice singing his name, a deep sense of emotional awareness and connectedness to himself emerged. He said that his name was not irritating to him anymore because of my singing. Often he commented that my voice was like silver, would calm him, take him out of his mood, influence his emotions and help him to relax. He especially talked about the effect of my voice, not the musical actions, comforting him. My approach required sensitive vocal shifts, because when Paul was experiencing great pain, he panicked, thought that he was dying and uttered primal sounds. He could only survive in bed with strong medication. No jokes, songs or other intellectual conversation would calm him. In this condition, I would sing to him, not familiar songs but relaxing improvised sounds and words. His fear was still so intense that he reacted to every strong cognitive intervention. Telling me about his fear, he buried his face in the pillows and was anxious about dying. At those moments I switched to nonverbal vocal sounds, no words, no instruments, no diversionary tactics. I did not go to the physical level of his pain but affectively transformed his acoustic symbols into a neurological effect.

I attempted a trusting and comforting contact through soft whispering or smooth vocal sounds, like long "ahhh's" in a centric melodic form and simple rhythm. Using only my natural vibrato or none at all, connecting myself to his breath, singing and humming softly with an airy sound, after a few minutes Paul stopped fussing and started relaxing. While I was singing open vocal sounds, a simple ostinato pattern like a lullaby without words, he fell asleep and with that the pain left him. I experienced his fearful disorientation as a serious condition like the coma and offered a primal vocal comfort with a maternal approach.

On the **technical level** my improvisations were simple: a cappella, or I repeated two chords on my keyboard, or moved from a song melody to an improvisation using its chord progression, for example F/Am/C/G/Em. I mostly used major progressions to avoid more sad feelings and sometimes combined them with minor tonalities. When I wanted to soothe him I also used the sound of strings on the keyboard to increase the relaxation effect through long tones.

Paul's favourite song was "Somewhere over the Rainbow"; this was his escape-song, he said. Often he requested it and I sang this song because it "relieved whatever was hurting him," he said. I sang low and high between F and F2, mostly in the original key. Sometimes I sang with full-bodied voice which had the effect of making him look at me as if I was his personal performer. I was aware when I had to sing with a performing voice or a nurturing maternal sound, consciously using more or less body support.

On the **spiritual level,** singing to him while he was in pain in his bed, I fully transcended my sound into conscious vibration, changing from doing into being the sound. My theoretical familiarity and experiences of spiritual training supplied in those moments the transition into trance. Sometimes Paul acted as if he was my audience in a concert hall and he treated me thankfully when I was singing only for him. He often was emotional and gave me compliments as if he were in love with me, blowing kisses and giving me charming smiles. Being aware of his transference, my singing might have expanded his level of experience, changed place and time for him and at times enabled him to enter into a light trance state. Maybe he reached a different level of consciousness that 'relieved whatever was hurting him,' as he said.

The **physical level** was touched when I was standing in front of Paul's bed, focusing on my position and direction of sound. Acknowledging cultural traditions with awareness of sound vibration and the different directions in nature, his position in the wheelchair awoke my attention through its limited receptivity. Attuning myself to body-centered vocalization, sometimes walking around his wheelchair while singing, I tried to reach him through non-forced singing and free vibration, acknowledging the neurological response to my frequencies. Observing Paul's body patterns and paralysed parts I directed my sound into those areas. The resonance and effect of my own sound was intensely dependent on my level of relaxation or tension, and I attuned myself to my own inner resources. Through this vibration I tried to connect him with himself, with his environment and myself, reaching out to something bigger than him.

Accepting and interacting with Paul's sarcastic comments as well as painful sounds, his shadow connected me to the **aesthetic level** of our work. His limited sound, yawning, painful mourning and his harsh sarcasm about himself and his environment touched me personally. I learned to appreciate his authentic sounds, and imitated, adapted or commended them through being in dialogue with him. I made those sounds transparent to his own inner world and comforted him vocally, interacting from 'one human howl to another.' He profoundly appreciated the comfort and relaxation he attained and he asked me to make a recording of our work, so he could use it when I was not available.

Wanting to fully understand the depth of his response, I studied his answers to the effect of my treatment. With Paul I was able to communicate verbally. Using a scale from 1-10, after every session he noted if his feelings of well-being had improved. Whatever condition he started in, the vocal intervention enhanced his well-being between 2 and 9 levels. This treatment was also directly effective in lowering his blood pressure each time. I could vocally calm him and bring tiny moments of peace into his life. I could not cure his illness, but I embraced his lonely fear and confusion into my understanding and serene sound, improving his quality of life. My simple melodic, repetitive vocalizations as well as my songs interacted with his needs. I adapted and integrated his acoustic symbols into a vital consciousness in this cold medical setting, sharing sound and silence with him. I have learned through working this way that singing may be the most direct and effective caring instrument for this kind of treatment. I also have learned to profoundly differentiate between the qualities of my voice, realizing when I had to switch or to stop using it.

This example of my own therapeutic singing, and the methods and techniques I have developed through my personal and clinical work, give conclusive evidence of the living tradition of healing self and others through authentic vocal expression.

INTERMEZZO

This switch, leaving my personal and clinical material, going to an anthropological observation about different vocal cultures, seems to be a profound change. For readers not interested in detailed information about other cultures (as described in Part B), please feel free to go to Part C where practical voice workshop information includes some clinical and multi-cultural thoughts. Meanwhile with the following part of this book I'd like first to support my personal and clinical work, and second to open our ears to universal voices.

Part B of this book highlights traditional forms of authentic singing in cultural perspective. From all over the world I've gathered knowledge and experience in the numerous ways of human vocal expression used to help and heal. Here, by means of examples of age-old practices from different continents, the treasures of primitive singing–meaning purely the natural, authentic source of original sound–are detailed. Some of these vocal treasures are nearly forgotten and are presented now to preserve their richness and to remind us where our authentic vocal expressions have their roots.

In the following chapters we explore a unique world of vocal expressions including examples from African slaves, Kurdish mourners and Native American healers, and many other global voices. With this collection of primitive music as well as cultivated singing traditions, I mirror the universal human behaviour of spontaneously and naturally expressing emotions and thoughts through authentic singing. Such authentic forms of singing in different cultures are distinguished by their functions, for example, as serving productive, spiritual or survival purposes. Often such functions overlap. To differentiate their characteristics I focus on the primary function. For example, in Kurdish culture the individual vocal improvisations about sorrow in front of their houses, under a tree or in a cemetery, is a typical expression of grief. This archetype of individual vocal expression also has collective benefits. And the collective singing of Native Americans, for example as community healing, also offers individual consolation. Both are good examples for us to learn from in order to understand that individual singing has collective effects and vice versa. Both are authentic arts of vocal expression, and together with other traditions, form a body of primitive, authentic singing, rich in cultural aspects of healing and functioning for the community. Awareness of myriad perspectives will broaden our curiosity about the voice and any psychotherapeutic approach will only be enhanced through a multicultural understanding.

PART B

AUTHENTIC SINGING

Chapter VIII

Vocal sound in primitive expression and functions of singing are evaluated in this chapter in terms of productive, healing and ritualistic practices with special emphasis on the role of the female voice. In *Primitive Singing* I expound on Otto Karolyi's thoughts on how vocal expression brings chaos into new order and helps primitive feelings to organize and to transform. Through *Productive Singing* I contrast Karl Adamek's modern research on the enormous power of energizing vocalizations with the survival of Negro productive song tradition through a rich history. In *Ritualistic Singing* I describe how according to Françoise O'Kane rituals function so that psychic contents get projected onto nature and social environment. The image of nature as being both 'nourishing and cruel' comprises a practical analogy for human beings for their transformation process through the voice. Multicultural examples illustrate vocal practices in shamanistic rituals while *Female Singing* depicts the practice of myriad female healing voices. Through Annette Cramer's explanation of female wisdom and Holst-Warhaft's specialty of female lament, the power of female voices and their significance in history becomes clear and perhaps implies that the female voice terrified some cultures.

PRIMITIVE SINGING

In the research on vocal sounds and theories of the common origin of speech and music, the roots for authentic vocalizations are debatable. Karolyi (1998) quotes Darwin's thought of its origin in the imitation of "lone cries during the mating season" and Rousseau's proposal of "speech as a form of song" outlining the controversy. Although the origin of speech and music is so controversial, the idea of a transforming function is obvious. Karolyi, teacher and writer about Western and non-Western music, states that music seems to have the power to direct the highly subjective and personal towards the objective and universal. He clarifies this power with the belief that it is easier to sing a love song rather than announce words of love. And thoughts set to music are more proper, more general or ambiguous than those thoughts expressed in words alone. The difference is that the thought becomes a theme to a regular rhythm, a structured form.

In the Mediterranean area of Europe, for example, the tradition of the narrative epic song is still alive. Putting words to a regular rhythm, called the art of bardic verse, is a valid medium today. This tradition helps us to understand how this art would have been practiced in the ancient world and to learn about its benefits. Bardic verse must have been the first vocal expression of the Homeric epics, rooted in its Greek history and carrying and expressing centuries of history into our times in forms of poetic composition. Here I see a connection between the ancient and the contemporary use of improvised singing. I found an interesting reflection about vocal traditions in Karolyi's interpretation of African music:

> Vocal music can be regarded as an expression in its own right. The spontaneity of expression is made apparent by often speechlike (recitative) style mixed with the song, as if the word were helping to find the music and vice versa. Pygmy performers often start with wild shouts. Out of these inarticulate articulations slowly the music is born, as if a journey were to be taken from chaos to order and from the personal to a communal harmony (Karolyi, 1998, p. 20).

I surmise that Karolyi's explanation about simple vocal expression can be expanded beyond African music to describe a general fact that through spontaneous vocalization with words alone improvised to a regular rhythm, chaos grows into order. This idea of chaos into order is also used by Wilber as a principle in his thoughts of evolution. Wilber gives philosophical justification to the inherent limitations of development of the world through a type of chaos. During chaos the old system breaks down in a form of self-dissolution or escapes this chaos by evolving to a higher degree of order, a form of self-transcendence. The order out of chaos evolution is rooted in those thoughts; this new order breaks away from the limitations of its ancestor.

If I apply those thoughts of chaos into order to everyday life, I rediscover the need for a personal evolution: having breakdowns and burnouts, being in dissolution or escaping the limitations of yesterday and moving to a higher degree of order, being transcendent. As complicated or difficult to achieve this may seem in daily life, the primitive art of singing perhaps brings us to this experience of higher order most quickly and directly, not only in African culture but everywhere. Satisfying the requirements of our personal evolution we look for transcendent forms of regeneration and contact; authentic singing can move us out of this chaos into a new order.

Many cultures have lost their natural forms of regeneration in their evolutionary process. Singing traditions are dying and with them the healing behaviour of transcendence. But also new tendencies appear to re-learn or re-integrate singing and its functional tradition. The famed sound scientist Dr. Alfred Tomatis was called to a Benedictine monastery in France to find a solution to an emerging problem among the monks. Accustomed to chanting their Gregorian chants for several hours daily, Tomatis discovered that when this routine was abolished, the monks became "listless, fatigued and mildly depressed." Tomatis determined that singing for twenty minutes nine times a day with intensive breathing had lowered their blood pressure and raised their moods and productivity. He solved the problem through his advice of continuing the ancient pattern of singing. After six months on a regular singing schedule, the monks were more healthy, delighted and productive.

PRODUCTIVE SINGING

Adamek wrote a book about daily singing and its function as a new/old way of helping ourselves in our modern time. Around the world, healthcare systems are not complete enough to cover all of the peoples' needs. At this time, when economics are dominating healthcare options, we need simple and effective ways for self-help. Adamek did many years of empirical research about how to use singing for your Self–with your authentic voice and not singing for an audience–as an aid to health and wellness. Here again we find the chaos-into-order transformation through singing. Adamek explained that singing helps people cope with myriad issues: sorting out basic personal questions, increasing concentration and learning, soothing depressive mood episodes, stimulating development, and especially, easing mental and emotional pain such as grief, loneliness, disappointment, sadness, desperation, world-weariness, trouble, yearning and homesickness.

In one of his research studies Adamek put weights onto the stretched arms of two groups of healthy students. While one group was singing and the other not, both groups held the weights up as long as possible. He discovered that the singers with weights were able to keep their arms stretched 5 minutes longer than those who were not singing. This example leads us to the function of work songs, used in labour, military, slave or concentration camps, to energize workers, soldiers or prisoners. Through coordinating the rhythm of the song with the work rhythm, productivity increased.

Negro songs often originate from songs of the slaves and illustrate how work songs function. These songs structured the labour and helped the slaves to stay alive despite their treatment. In a book about slave songs from 1867 these songs are also called "a breath of trusting faith," a breath of hope. Singing, improvising and shouting together, while they "hoisted and lowered the hogsheads and boxes of their cargoes," one man takes the burden of the song and the others strike in with the chorus. Here again is the chaos into order principle: getting in touch with the feelings and directly transforming them into a new form. Singing perhaps a "dozen different songs in one hour, innocent in their language, nothing religious but attractive in their music, their vocal volume reached a square or two away." Here is another taste from this book with its antique language to characterize the use of this effective singing style.[31]

> There is no singing in parts, as we understand it, and yet no two appear to be singing the same thing–the leading singer starts the words of each verse, often improvising, and the others, who 'base' him, as it is called, strike in with the refrain, or even join in the solo, when the words are familiar. When the 'base' begins, the leader often stops, leaving the rest of his words to be guessed at, or it may be they are taken up by one of the other singers. And the 'basers' themselves seem to follow their own whims, beginning when they please and leaving off when they please, striking an octave above or below . . . or hitting some other note that chords, so as to produce the effect of a marvellous complication and variety, and yet with the most perfect time, and rarely with any discord. And what makes it all the harder to unravel a thread of melody out of this strange network is that, like birds, they seem not infrequently to strike sounds that cannot be precisely represented by the gamut, and abound in 'slides from one note to another, and turns and cadences not in articulated notes.' . . . The odd turns made in the throat, and the curious rhythmic effect produced by single voices chiming in at different irregular intervals, seem almost as impossible to place on the score as the singing of birds or the tones of an Aeolian Harp (Allen, Ware & Garrison, p. V).

This singing style symbolizes the special sound quality of the Negro song. Rooted in the need of vocal expression as a form of survival, their voices are authentic. There is a peculiar vocal quality that nothing and nobody can imitate; even intonations and delicate variations cannot be reproduced. Their shouts described in this book as "runnin sperichils" (spirituals), distinguished from the other "sperichils," may appear to any tune and purpose. Perhaps the use of shouts is a relic of some native African dance and music. Thinking of the

---

31. This quote of a slaveholder shows his admiration as well as his disrespect for the authentic singing skills of his slaves: "The high voices, all in unison, and the admirable time and true accent with which their responses are made, always make me wish that some great musical composer could hear these semi-savage performances. With a very little skilful adaptation and instrumentation, I think one or two barbaric chants and choruses might be evoked from them that would make the fortune of an opera." (Mrs. Kemble, from "A Life on a Georgian Plantation" in Allen, Ware & Garrison 1867, *Slave Songs*, p. V.)

African vocal music described above, perhaps its spontaneous expression made often in speech-like or recitative style, was specified with some wild shouts. Shouts seen as inarticulate expressions are creating a new order, from the personal sound to a form of communal harmony. These shouts are heard on Sundays or on prayer nights throughout the week. Both songs and dances are extremely energetic; often, when the shouts last into the middle of the night, "the monotonous thud, thud of the feet prevents sleep within half a mile of the praise-house."

Technically it seems that hymns, songs and phrases were kept exquisite in rhythmical time; while singing and adapting words the slaves would force words or snatches into any duty with any tune they pleased. Through this it is understandable that the same songs were used for rowing as for shouting, inside and outside of the church. A pure boat-song and real spiritual is "Michael Row the Boat Ashore." Rhythmical shouting and singing during rowing was extremely effective. "Two measures are sung to each stroke, the first measure being accented by the beginning of the stroke, the second by the rattle of the oars in the rowlocks." Those songs without obvious words or messages but clear tone and melody set to a regular rhythm had an accommodating effect on the rowers. A slave trader was offering his own surprise about the veritable energetic result of the songs:

> But whatever may have been its real character [of the song], it was quite musical, and had such an inspiring effect upon my boatmen that I have known them to row eighteen or twenty miles, exerting their utmost strength, keeping perfect time to its notes, and never pausing for breath (pp. 115).

Negro songs were composed unexpectedly, often unconsciously made up at moments of need, putting words into a regular rhythm. "Some good sperituals are start jess out o' curiosity. Den I made a sing, just puttin' a word, and den anudder word." When this unknown composer started singing, the other men, after listening, joined in the chorus as if it was a known song. Learning about how the primitive songs were created helps me understand why they were so effective. When slaves were ordered to perform a tough job, their friends heard about it and felt sorry for their hardship. Meeting that night in the praise-house or outside, they would genuinely sing about it. Some great singers worked this one phrase into song, set words to a regular rhythm, improvised and finally produced a new song, as if a journey were to be taken from chaos into order and from the personal to a communal harmony, as described above. This archetypal function of transforming personal to communal harmony through vocalizations seems to be a universal, productive habit, often performed in ritualistic and healing forms.

RITUALISTIC SINGING

Rituals are established or prescribed procedures, systems, forms, ceremonies, services for religious or other rites, or codes of behaviour. There are more kinds of rituals than there are cultures, languages and dialects in this world, and each ritual has its own special role for music. In most forms of ritual, the voice and musical instruments have significant functions.

In the majority of indigenous cultures, the voice is typically an integral part of a ritual with a utilitarian magical, symbolic or social function within this oral tradition. The *Encyclopedia of Music* describes the role of the musician in the ritual:

> As an officiating member in a rite, the musician will be obliged to make his voice conform to a precise timbre and use it with a special technique determined by the circumstances. Sometimes he will give greater importance to voice production than to words themselves. . . . The shaman informs his hearers of the arrival of the spirit by a pronounced change in rhythm in his drum playing (Larousse, 1987, p. 17).

The significant role of the voice in ritual to heal sicknesses was often the secured practice of chosen individuals of communities, such as priests and doctors, helping others to transform chaos (illness) into order. Whether they were medicine persons, shamans and witches or mysterious doctors, the major similarity between these was the task of the human voice in the therapeutic process (see Chapter VIII, *Female Singing*).

The voice seems to have the outstanding role of transmitting the ritual's messages supported only by simple instruments. The voice and the drum are used to incarnate spirits, which distort their simple timbres. The healing effect develops through a large range of vocal sound techniques: strange timbres and cacophonies to personify evil spirits; recalling souls through vocal noise, screeches and improvised sonic forms; crying out or shouting regrets, touching the chaos inside and outside. The voice might take on a harsh grating sound, the registers becoming rapidly opposed, as experienced in yodeling, and the imitation of animal cries is very typical.

> In addition to formal ritual, singing holds some magical elements in songs for the "tilling of the soil, . . . songs to the oxen [or other animals] . . . ornate recitative chants with free rhythms . . . weeping psalmodising . . . chants, delivered at full

> voice into space, frequently end in rising scales or ascending cries" (p. 18).

The singing or noise-making voice, together with a kind of monotonous drum rhythm, build up the foundation for relaxing into or awakening an altered state of consciousness. The belief in a spiritual cause for illness helped the people in their attempt to connect themselves to a spiritual power affiliated with this altered state. It was believed that this power could be transmitted through the sound vibrations of the voice (see Chapter VI).

Francoise O'Kane (1994), a Jungian ethnologist and anthropologist, writes about the transformational role of rituals. "Ritual work structures the chaos of being and thus modifies it, rendering it more accessible," she says of primitive rituals in her book, *Sacred Chaos*. They might be understood as a form of projection: "psychic contents are projected onto nature and the social environment." Through ceremonies of ritual, individual or collective themes are confronted externally, but experienced deeply personally on physical, emotional, spiritual and social levels. The image of nature as being both 'nourishing and cruel' comprises a practical analogy for human beings for their transformation.

> Nature is just what it is, and encompasses the two poles, positive and negative, life and death, transformation and destruction. In that sense, those religions which attribute a central importance to the relationship between man and nature may serve as a model for defining the propitious attitude toward the duality of the Self (p. 36).

It could be possible to conclude that those who are in closer contact with nature and its changes and dualities might find it easier to touch, complete or transform their own Self. By using the transcendent function of ritual as a tool to discover the synthesis between good and evil, order and chaos, we express the true nature of the Self and unleash its healing capacities. The potential for healing emerges from our ability to include and transform, through the harsh grating sounds of a human voice, the paradoxes and contradictions of existence, such as evil and chaos and our shadow nature. The ritualistic processes of imagination, connection and communication help us to transcend individual experience, duality, and linear time, and ground us in the presence of nature and being.

The female personification of the witch has, through the centuries, illustrated the archetype of transcendence. The word *witch* originates from the German word for 'Hexe,' derived from 'Hecke' meaning hedge–the witch was 'the one who rides across the hedge.' She was the one who could 'ride' or communicate between two worlds. O'Kane describes the witch not only as the symbol of the negative mother but also as a symbol of liberation:

> [The witch] frees psychic energies and helps reorientate them. . . . [T]he witch often symbolizes a compensatory attitude which the psyche requires in order to free itself from the behavioral mechanism and one-sided ego choices that have contributed to a blockage of libido (O'Kane, p. 69).

Stories, movies and fairy tales all over the world depict witches with herbs and bizarre sounding voices, and especially with extremely powerful, dangerous laughter. Witches practice magic rituals, mediating between life and death, health and illness, their voices uttering socially unacceptable, or at least strange and often scary, sounds. Their intimidating power may perhaps start off from their untouchable, sensitive connection to nature. Might the fear of witches derive from their unique vocal ability to free themselves, as O'Kane described above, or touch chaos? This typical connection of the voice as an integral part of a ritual, which frees up energy with a utilitarian magical purpose, could drive the action of transcendence. Within shamanism the act of spiritual ritualistic healing combined with magical functions was once a worldwide phenomenon[32]. A shaman, using vocal sounds, dance, music and herbs, was able to connect with spirits, transcending into other dimensions. Both witches and shamans are believed to have the power to turn themselves into other spiritual creatures. In general it is thought that witches have bad spirits and can cause illness or death to their enemies, while shamans have the healing power to bond human beings to life.

Both men and women shamans were trained to treat the body and soul of a sick person and often reconnected them with a kind of superhuman power. The shaman was the power-connector, often dressed in women's clothes, reaching out into forms of female qualities and trance, working against witchcraft and bad spirits.

The shaman had the role of initiating and accompanying the person in a process called spiritual exorcism. This is how the shaman helps drive the evil out of the sick patient, similar to the process of catharsis. The patient is liberated

---

32. I also want to mention African music again, the role model for the vocal music I described above. Original African shamanic healing traditions became strongly modified by other religions. Typical for all African music is the role of the singing voice with the preference for collective rather than individual song, and the prominence of the polyphonic. Also involved is the use of quick delivery of texts, explosive sounds or particular interjections, vocal grunts, as well as whispers. As I described in the examples of slave songs, during work, in mourning or ordinary pray rituals in the church shouting is typical; one "takes over the singing when the church members rejoice in the spirit. Rejoicing is accompanied by rhythmic vocalizations which are singular and movingly beautiful" (Cook, 1997, p. 48).

of poisonous and violating spirits and emotions and is thereby decontaminated. The role of the voice in this process can be entirely different from the ordinary singing voice. The healer's role as an active participant in the process is central in shamanic tradition. Sometimes the healer takes parts of the evil spirits from the patient into his own body (getting in touch with chaos), and later drives them out through self-exorcism (transforming it into a new order).

Shamanism is a healing art still practiced in small communities all over the world, from Central Asia to Central America. Communicating with animals, spirits and human beings through singing and playing is essential in their work[33]. A Peruvian Ayahuasca Shaman from the Amazon River, for example, believes that the spirit is doing the healing: "I am simply a middleman," he says. The songs he uses in his work are extraordinary and they "can cause listeners to vomit, cry, scream and experience any other mental or bodily effect." He believes that the "cries are very important because they help rid you of things that have been buried there for many years, from tragedies. Tears and the combination of songs with herbs penetrating the stomach and caus[ing] vomiting, works for him to release toxins and oxidants" (Cook, 1997, p. 23). (See Appendix B for more examples.)

As the above examples demonstrate, the significance of crying, singing, shouting or explosive sounds, as well as the intense contact with nature, is that these transmit the human being into the contact with one's Self and its surroundings. In general, I conclude that while the drum of the Shaman has the role of transporting him to different places, the voice has the role of connecting with the power of the animals through the phenomena of vocal noise, overtones, phonation and phraseology. This connection seems to be extremely powerful with its healing effect in shamanistic, ritualistic traditions. The power of being taken from chaos into order and from the personal to a communal harmony forms the theme in the following examples and traditions too.

FEMALE SINGING

It seems that many cultures have preserved the original tradition of spontaneous breaking into songs of support, grief, lamenting, sing-crying or shouting. Thinking of the job working men had to perform during tough labour, women often supported their men mentally and emotionally. The songs of the slaves were preserved through cultural roles: men noticeable outside the house,

---

33. In *The Story Of The Weeping Camel*, a documentary made by THINKFilm and National Geographic World Film, a Mongolianshaman, for example, uses music to melt the heart of a camel that had rejected her newborn.

working together and listening to each other's songs; women inside the house, also sharing their invisible hardship and emotions through songs. Surprisingly, through history the role of the earliest artist and healer was considered to be female, as I will describe in the following examples.

There are different ways to think about the female singing role. It is possible that from the popularity of the 'singing slave girls' (qaynas), the role of the female entertainer as performing musician emanated from the Arabic world, as Karolyi mentioned. But this role goes far beyond entertainment because the original healers all around the world were often singing women, medicine women, magicians, sorcerers, witch-doctors, lamenters, or shamans.

The female power of inspiring wisdom came from the ancient tradition of female healers, a tradition where the male was subordinate. The role as healer/artist in the dynasty of Ur (ca. 2500 BC) for example, showed female musicians strongly connected to their kings, sharing their death and following them even to the grave. Music seemed to be extremely important, not only during life but also through dying and death. Many early pictures and poems show females from Mesopotamia to China as artists, priests and healers practicing mystic and rational therapies. Mystic forms were the respected form of therapy, performed by the female priest-doctor, using sacred words and rituals. Rational therapy was the more profane medical and chirurgical form. Chirurgic treatment was simply compared with craftsmanship.

Being connected to a source of wisdom, women used their authentic voices for healing through wise sayings, singing and sacred rituals. Female mouths were time and again exhibited as the mouth of their sex organs. This is the gate for the breath of life as well the breath of speech. The life of every human being starts at this point, and assuming the connection of the sex organs with the speaking mouth, both are giving birth to vital life. Herein lies the female power of producing verbal and organic life. The name of the Indian God Vac means language, speech coming out of a mouth. But it could imply a further connection to vagina, the opening of the female sex organ. This Indian God Vac is pictured as motherly opening of the mouth, often symbolized for the double interpretation (Cramer).

Starting around 10,000 BC in the East and West, female power in cultures around the world was first established through monotheism[34] where many societies revered a Great Mother. Following Wilber's thought about the relationship between men and women, both were equal and were involved in the agricultural production of food. Then the distinguishing processes of separation appeared between women working at home protecting their pregnancies and preventing miscarriages, caused largely through hard work in the fields, and men conscripted for defence and agrarian work. Because of this new position of

34. Monotheism is the belief that there is only one God.

men as food producers, the deity figures switched from female-oriented to male-oriented. Wilber uses the example: "Where females work the field with a hoe, God is a Woman; where males work the field with a plow, God is a Man." (p. 51) This evolutionary progression toward patriarchy subordinated women from around 4000-2000 BC. Men specialized from food production into new technologies and science; women stayed with the reproductive forms. From this time on men tried to protect themselves from the previous supremacy of women. Through religion and culture, males dominated females and more and more silenced women through law and order.

The loss of these women's voices as vehicles for expressing personal as well as communal grief has its echo in our cultures today. The dangerous and unknown power of female witches and shamans were often enough related to madness and so these women were simply executed. The energy of uncontrollable emotional power is dangerous for the one who cannot experience it. Being able to touch chaos and possibly transform it is powerful. The similarity to disorderly psychic stages of mind classified in psychiatric illness is not difficult to see. Women in the past were easily diagnosed as 'hysterical' when their mysterious expressions were actually rooted in the emotional quality of life, a concept that was too foreign for the rational thinking of the time.

Besides their equality as workers, the major influence of women throughout history has been the supremacy of their powerful authentic voices. This authority was hidden as through the centuries women, held as unequal, were concealed, suppressed and governed. Women stayed in the home and became the caretakers of personal and social life. The practice of performing laments or spontaneous breaking into forms of song survived in some cultures and women clearly became the self-appointed mourners, not only of death. To compose, sing and express grief, rage, compassion or mysticism through music, was the practice of women as the sensors of human life. And Wilber challenges our new spirituality when he says:

> And one of the great tasks of spirituality in the postmodern world is to complement and balance this male-oriented spirituality with its correlative female forms (p. 55).

It is interesting to point out that when men are not the primary producers and defenders anymore, their average life expectancy increases to match that of women (Ghiglieri). By sharing responsibilities the liberation will be equal, and men will know that they benefit from it. The emancipation of women conveys already more equality and responsibility, but with the result that the female voice has changed into lower, more masculine sounds (see Chapter VI) but is unable yet to access its feminine spirit and earlier supreme wisdom.

Female voice qualities vary strongly through storytelling, laments, lullabies and healing songs. The values of female voices are transformative, obliging and comforting. In one cross-cultural example, females use ordinary, social laughter more than twice as much as men throughout any conversation. And laughter in general has a disarming, maybe ingratiating effect. It seems to work more as a 'contagious social lubricant' says Ghiglieri (1999) in his book *The Dark Side of Man*. When we hear somebody laughing, often we laugh too and generally feel better after that. If men would like to raise their life expectancy closer to that of females, they should join them in laughing, crying and perhaps authentic singing.

In the earliest times of pre-Islamic periods, women had the prominent roles of singers and healers, musicians, dancers and composers, as in the Kurdish tradition I will describe later. In the ancient Christian Greek and Irish traditions there were scores of rituals performed by women. The lament, for example, articulated "elaborate poems to tuneful weeping" about death. Holst-Warhaft (1992), in her book *Dangerous Voices*, explains women's laments, called "moiroloi," as coming from the Greek root mora=fate and logos=speech, or word. She describes the prominent role of women in the mourning ritual and the difference from men. She also talks about the uneasiness by men in many cultures where laments are generally performed by women (for example, China, New Guinea, India, rural Greece and Italy, Finland and the Bedouin of Saudi Arabia).

Women carried out the dominant role in the rituals of death as well as birth mostly in the villages. Holst-Warhaft explains that in societies where most of the deaths were children, it was 'natural' that the mothers were the ones caring for them from birth to death. The aspect of expressing their pain through their voices through weeping, or sing-crying, could be developed as a song form that was directly addressed to the deceased. Herein lies the cradle of the authentic singing, articulating the feelings of the moment: laments were made to inform members of the family or a small community that the dead are missed.

But laments were also sung in some cultures on other occasions to mediate between life and death. The threat of death is reduced when during weddings, for example, a lament is sung while brides are leaving their homes. Departure and separation from the protection of the well-known environment of the parents' home seems to be a little death for the girl, and singing a lament gives the impression of relief and comfort for the tears.

There are differences between man and woman in the way they mourn. Bedouin men, for example, do not cry, but if necessary they weep silently; otherwise they refer to the will and mercy of God if someone dies. An exception is when Bedouin men are 'singing' poems in a quivering voice during the annual festival at the tombs of saints. Going around from tent to tent, they bless for respect and curse for disrespect; this singing sounds exactly like the crying over the saint. These sounds are approved for men in a ceremonial context, but not in a private one.One could infer that the embarrassment of crying for men created emotional freedom for women. There was nothing to lose because–in the majority of 78 cultures researched, from Finland to New Guinea–women expressed pain and grief more than men. So women became the manipulator of the magical language of lament, representing bridges between life and death. Despite being oppressed by later patriarchal societies, they became influential with death, touching the untouchable fear of chaos in humans.

Holst-Warhaft claimed that this kind of dialogue with the dead gave women a special power, which was effective especially in societies where blood feuds were expressed by the violent rhetoric of funeral laments. Women's power is supposed to arouse the dead to revisit the living or to take revenge:

> It is not simply saying that men and women mourn differently, but that one is better than the other, especially in the context of a funeral of a man who dies . . . a hero. A hero's death, it seems, should be marked by praise, not women's cries, that may 'wake the dead.' If their cries have such power, women must be capable of some direct communication with the dead (p. 2).

One major difference between men and women is in the depth and freedom of the vocal language of pain. Women are weeping longer and louder, with more varieties of timbre, pitch, sobs, moans, shrieks and sighs and they are finally able, maybe on an unconscious level, to get in touch with the dead. For men in most cultures it would be dishonourable to cry loud out. Instead there is often a connection made to the glory of dying for the fatherland or some other honoured service. These correlations often compensate men for their loss.

In most cultures it has been women, not men, who have broken into songs of grief. Additionally these laments can even evolve from songs of grief to songs of anger or ecstatic revenge. It's easy to imagine how this might be threatening to men. Consciously or unconsciously, the female skill of transforming emotion out of chaos, bewilderment or grief into a new order creates empowerment. Especially in occupied territories such as Ireland and Palestine/Israel the laments have sometimes transformed into revenge. It has fired men to break out into war and focus on the male side of grief: anger. Anger seems to be the only emotion where men exceed women in the emotional depth of their answer.

Holst-Warhaft goes back in history to the Byzantine period and comments that women, maybe against the state in antiquity and the Christian church, continued "to be the self-appointed mourners of the death, composing and singing laments to express their grief and often their rage at losing their loved ones."

Fear of death in Western or Modern societies, with its hospitalisations and medicalisations, causes us to avoid discourses with death as a part of life and makes mourning rituals meaningless. The echoes of women's laments contribute to the poetic art of any society where the vocal village tradition is still alive to preserve the ritualistic language of death. The only surviving manifestation of lament in the West–as language of the death–seems to be the Blues. With its roots in the folk tradition, the Blues keep alive the language of grief and especially also the rage of the living in the face of death.

The vocal power of getting in touch with the untouchable, the dark side in us–in temporary as in historical time–creates the potential for healing grief, misery or illness[35]. The life of every human being starts and ends at this point, and remembering the connection of the sex organs with the speaking mouth, this is the point where healing can rise. Being able to touch fear, illness, suffering, spirits, death and life; women were empowered by their self-healing instruments.

I am closing these thoughts about mysterious inarticulate articulations of humans, as if a journey were to be taken from chaos into order and from the personal to a communal harmony. Creating songs has often been a part of bearing and surviving the poverty of life. Slaves sang gravely during tough work, easing their lives through the energy generated by the voice. Also singing as energy-integrator for channelling emotional energy, changing moods, affecting our minds and bodies, as the meditative chants of the French monks and the lament rituals around the world, has been shown to be highly effective. In many Western traditions daily singing is slowly disappearing and there is increasing need to learn from other cultures where the desire to sing still exists: singing alone as an important component of the day, and sharing it through rituals within their community.

---

35. See M. Gaynor M.D.'s book, The Healing Power of Sound, which describes the potential to recover from cancer and life-threatening illness while using sound, voice and music.

Chapter IX

With examples from the Middle East, in this chapter I illustrate the existing tradition of improvised singing through various individual, spiritual and religious practices. *Middle Eastern-Kurdish Singing* delineates the historical and political condition of Kurdish people to express their needs and suffering through songs. In *Improvisational Singing* I describe the Kurdish spontaneous singing and composing tradition–improvising a singing newspaper with therapeutic effect. *Spiritual Singing* offers a glance at Kurdish Sufi ritual, performed by industrialized spiritual adults in Western country. While *Islamic "Singing"* forms call out for the name of God, its orthodox tradition does not change its hostility about music; singing and performing is too intensely sensitive, questioning the morale of the musicians. But Güvenç's holistic old-oriental music therapy approach reaches far into history. At more than a thousand years old, this therapeutic approach to connect body and soul through music is one of the first of its kind. While various Islamic animated folk music traditions from North Africa and Afghanistan survive until today, their mostly female composers are invisible and unknown.

MIDDLE EASTERN–KURDISH SINGING

Kurdish culture is one of the cultures that still maintains the tradition of original improvised singing. I deliberately want to use the example of an ancient culture with a strong individual vocal and improvisational tradition for expressing pain, grief and loss. I hope to explore with this the archetype of primitive individual singing in ancient and contemporary times and its importance for therapeutic use. Music was and is able to transcend time and geographical distance as well as to resolve political quarrels, and can help to heal personal and historical wounds. I'd like to start with a brief introduction to the Kurdish culture to establish a context of the political and cultural aspects and specific problems.

Kurdistan, the land of the Kurds, in the center of the Middle East, inhabits parts of Turkey, Iran, Iraq, Syria, Armenia and Azerbaijan. The Kurdish language is Indo-European in origin, a branch of Indo-Iranian tongue (see Chapter IV, *Linguistic Voices*). As of today the independence of Kurdistan is still denied, and Kurds are the biggest minority in the world without their own country. The successive governments of Turkey, Iran, Iraq, Syria and the former Soviet Union are unable to offer a clear census of the Kurdish population. Counts vary widely, estimated at 30.5 million, with over half of these, 16.5

million, living in Turkey, 7.3 million in Iran, 4.7 million in Iraq, 1.4 million in Syria, 400,000 in former Soviet Union and 1 million in Europe, Israel, Lebanon, the USA and other parts of the world.

References to the name of the Kurds appear in history from 3000–400 BC. One of the oldest nations in the Middle East, the ancestors of the Kurds are the ancient Medes (from Media). Long periods of disturbances between Kurdistan and its neighbours, a history of invasions, massacres, language and culture denial, mark their identity. With the success of their immediate neighbours occupying their country, the Kurds as an ethnic minority were deprived of a national identity and artificially classified into the homogeny of those nations.[36]

The pain of this forced integration and denial of Kurdish identity is still expressed in their poems and songs containing especially sorrowful emotions. The musical tradition of the Kurds is deeply connected with the daily life of farmers or city dwellers; some music still tells about their original nomadic life, some about love, longing, exile, hope and sensuous nostalgia. And some Kurdish music is still devoted to songs which pay tribute to the valiant Peshmerga, the Kurdish resistance fighters in Iraq. For years the singers themselves could be imprisoned for singing these songs. Many Kurdish singers and musicians still live outside of Turkey, Iran, Iraq and Syria, unable to return home-but the conditions in those countries are changing. Empowered by performing songs abroad in their mother tongue, they still send delicate cultural and political messages out through their feelings and music. Several are still performing in their homelands, singing in the official languages of the countries they reside in, including only a few Kurdish songs in their repertoire.

For decades speaking and singing in Kurdish in Turkey resulted in imprisonment, denying the very existence of Kurds. Even at present, although there are no ongoing wars, and even with the easements for Kurdish language by the Turkish government as part of the EU-inspired reforms starting in 2004, there are still problems in practice for the free expression of Kurdish.

Countless songs of longing for homeland exist, speaking the language of tenderness and pain. The song "Homeland" by Xalid Rashid laments the soreness of the separation and longing for Kurdistan.

---

36. McDowall notes that seventy-five percent of the Kurds are Sunni Islamite. The rest follow ancient religions such as the Alevis (or Alevites) in central Anatolia, claiming devotion to Imam Ali (Imam Ali A.D. c.600-661, the fourth caliph for Sunnis, first Imam for Shia, cousin of Prophet Mohammed). The Alevi religion is a mixture of pre-Islamic, Zoroastrian, (Turkoman) Shamanism and Shi'i Islam, forming a religious sect in the fifteenth century CE. The Alevis of Kurdistan are mainly speakers of Dimili/Zaza dialect of Kurdish, spoken in the north of Turkey. The Ahl-e Haqq sect of southern Kurdistan (Kermanshah) speaks Gurani dialect of Kurdish.

O my homeland, I am sad and crying for you
O my homeland, I burn for your pain, for which I have no medicine.
O my homeland, I am your Jacob and I have lost my Joseph.
O my homeland, you have given me a bad name, and taken my integrity away.O my homeland, once you were a great nation,
When you were not in the hands of occupiers, not splintered as you are now.
O my homeland, the autumn will come; it will be my time.
The weather blowing warm and cold, like the moods of my divided heart.
Your wind is my sigh, your clouds are my eyes, the small rain that falls,
my suffering.

(Xalid Rashid, *Music from Kurdistan*)

IMPROVISATIONAL SINGING

Kurdish music belongs to the same group as Persian–not Arab–music. Kurdish music seems to be both a learned music and a folk music. Kurdish music is instinctive and impulsively passionate, sensuous, personal, refined and distinguished. The main characteristics of Middle Eastern music, including Kurdish, Persian and Arab, are its quasi-improvisational style and its foundation in and emphasis on vocals (see also Chapter XI). Because of the mainly oral tradition and official restrictions of governments there seems to be very little published about Kurdish music. However, one description is by the French ethnomusicologist Christian Poché, who describes this music supremely:

> The basic structure is a modal development upon which the elements are elaborated and organized by improvisation in such a way as to always result in a melodic-rhythmic conclusion. The music of the Kurds is strongly instinctive and impulsive and has great antiquity which has preserved its originality to the present day. In this tradition there is no precise term relating to the art of making music; the rules, the forms, the musical scales are in Kurdish language all associated with concrete phenomena. The basic notions are

expressed by simple terms taken from daily life and generalized (Poché).

To convey the idea of an improvisation the Kurds use a term that means 'work.' The improvisation in this culture is a basic aspect of the music; it reflects vocal and instrumental music. The musician has to work: to work at the lyrics, the contents and the melodies. The music, because of its intense improvisational character, produces songs with themes and incidents in the moment. Because of this construction Poché concluded that its function could be presented as the "healing of a wound" as in the moment of singing problems are worked out and coping is offered.

As discussed above, one of the general characteristics of Arab, Persian and Kurdish music is authentic vocal improvisation. The storyteller, or a popular epic singer, would never narrate the same story twice in the same way. Christensen studied Kurdish music traditions of regional cultures and the music-related behaviour and distinguished several categories that differ in use, function, structure and also variability. He found that only the epic singing exhibits "a very high degree of variability in the very same elements of music structure with all Kurdish groups studied." The capacity to create new lyrics for existing melodies or improvisations has been the most important skill for a singer in Kurdistan. The music is fundamentally based on monody, sung by a single voice, and is linear, which either takes the form of an austere, unadorned line or of a highly embroidered arabesque punctuated by vocalizations and improvisations. The melody is developed through intervals comprising a variety of tones and semitones and a great number of vocal timbres. Larousse portrayed these musical characters so, explaining that they give this music refined nuances and great expressive power.

From various sources I have learned that originally women were the authentic performers of the unadorned melodic line, simple or ornamented with arabesques and semitones. The Kurdish women in the villages transformed daily news into song lines through improvisation; they sat in front of their houses singing about their feelings of loss, pain, grief, and daily events using simple melodies and a great reservoir of vocal, emotional timbres. This music was absolutely different in its quality from the daytime music of festivities with its sharply accented rhythmic and melodic music. Only at night time did the musicians allow themselves moments of personal exultation, of withdrawal and of silence that contrasted with the 'noisy daytime music,' as Poché characterized this singing style.

The Kurds often use names of women, regions or tribes to denote a name for a mode or scale (maqam). When a maqam is called, for example, *maqam Mariame*, it means that it is in tribute to a particular melodic motif, given mostly through the ethos of the young woman Mariame. Songs called *gorani* are popular short and non-narrative forms found all over Kurdistan, easy to learn and having a refrain that appears to be longer than the verse. Dance, lyrical and political songs are identified as *gorani*, but many singers specialize in just one kind which determine the statuses for its performers. Night music with its improvisation called *Lawko,* meaning a beloved one, was sung in the mountains; while when sung in the plains, it was called *Lodelal,* meaning a way of singing. *Kirive* is a typical song about profound grief and passionate longing and the forbidden intermarriage between different religious groups.[37] The song demands the listener to overcome religious differences. Traditional and temporary love songs often symbolize the deep connection to the loved one and nature, and tell about adoration and the pain of longing, for example, "You are my cure."

All of these songs were vocally improvised personal expressions woven from existing songs There are still numerous different singing styles in Kurdish music and there is an enormous significance placed on the interpretation of these songs:

> You sing a song. . . . It is not the same thing at night and during the day. If a child sings a song, it is one thing, but when sung by a woman it will be something different, and it will also vary according as it is performed by young people or old people. A song is not the same in the mountains and in the plains, in the forest and at sea. It varies every time. In the morning, at noon, in the afternoon or the evening, it is not the same thing. (Kurdish musician quoted by Poché)

In the creation of this atmosphere of intimacy, the instruments used include the tanboura or kemenche (string instruments), the pik reed flutes, and above all the human voice. The musical structure is in the form of a primitive song; the music is simple and based solely on the use of one single mode. The characteristic of the Kurdish single mode is different from, for example, Indian music, which uses numbers of modes (more on this later). This bears witness to the antiquity of the Kurdish culture which has developed its tradition by preserving a single scale, known as the art of metabolism, meaning transposing within the mode. Through intense fluidity in the music, rooted on simple

---

37. In this song the girl tells about her love to somebody she cannot reach because of religious quarrels. She is telling the boy she loves about her mind's eye, how she feels about him and how her love is so strong that if they cannot be together only death remains for her. She relates herself to the gorgeous nature, the birds and gazelles of Kurdistan. She tells of her vulnerability in a situation outside her control. (Laizer, 1991, p. 40)

elements and developing various microtones, a rich complexity of sound can be established.

The typical mode of Kurdish music, a minor second followed by a major second, characterizes the maqam *'kord'* (or kurd; see Appendix A for the melodic structure of the scale). This is close to the Dorian mode employed by the Flamenco musicians of Spain. The similarity between the Dorian mode and the Kurdish scale is not so strange if we think of the origins of these musical styles. Flamenco comes from the Roma culture and has its roots in Rajasthan, Northern India, travelling from Asia through the Middle East to Europe.[38] Another connection to the Dorian mode could be the invasion of Hellas around 1200 BC, the same time range when the Medes (ancient Kurds) appeared. Both belong to Indo-European origin.

The idea of a concert is nearly unknown in Kurdish culture: music is made in any surrounding and at any time, by a group of friends seated round a table, under a tree, during a social evening or at home. In some areas of Iranian Kurdistan the listeners become performers themselves when "face-to-face encounters"[39] (Blum & Hassanpour) create a new act of music in response to the song. During social gatherings songs often have been able to bridge dialect and language barriers, spreading their music into different regions. The songs are mostly about village or rural life and later carried to the teahouses of cities. The songs have strophic structure and are generally constructed with two distinct melodic phrases, which correspond to the couplet and refrain. Some of the traditional Kurdish pieces are accompanied by dances; men and women form a circle which is led by a trained dancer who holds a scarf in his/her hand. The types of dances and the steps that make them up are varied and operate solely in relation to the measure of the rhythms and their accents (The Kamkars).

A Kurdish musician is above all a storyteller, even when s/he does not use any words or only poetry with symbolic imagery. But the wide range of human sentiment, the joyous and tragic love stories, the eternal struggle of human against nature, and the importance of tradition are communicated through their voices. The bards (called Dengbej) tell their stories which can continue for hours, legends which characteristically convey an emotion of sadness, and audience members are often seen to weep.

---

38. Throughout Central Asia, Eastern Europe, and along the Mediterranean, the Roma (Gypsies) have endured discrimination. They began their migration more than 1000 years ago. This incorporation of Roma and local traditions has created a rich and varied musical repertoire, rooted in elements popular among the Roma: vocal improvisations, rapid tempo changes, universal stories of life on the road, tragedies of lost love, and the dream of an era without discrimination (Rosenberg, 1999, CD cover).
39. The listener from audience gets his or her turn to sing.

> Sometimes the musician may even appear to function as a kind of healer who assuages the affections of the listener; the latter will seek out the musician and confide his problems to him: he may have lost the woman he loved, she may have abandoned him, or he may have fallen in love. He will sing and improvise until his listener is ready to depart in a soothed and relaxed mood. In such cases music acts as a form of social therapy (Christian Poché).

Rich vocal improvisations with numerous vocal timbres are an important factor in this emotional process of phrasing and overcoming pain. In this tradition, the singer, through storytelling, holds the significance of the message and has a strong impact on the listeners around him. Depending on the region where the musician lives, the spontaneous vocal exchange of emotional and private information and the communication about it with their environment is preserved through the voice as the cardinal instrument.

> Often it is a pure cry, without any instrumental accompaniment, a cry from the heart of a wounded beast. In Kurdistan one sings only of unhappy, unrequited love, and unusually for Islamic people, it is the woman who composes and sings the songs of love, at least within her own village or valley, before wandering minstrels–men–take up these songs and perform them on their travels (Institut Kurde, Paris).

As the ethnomusicologist Christian Poché said, and the Kurdish Institute in Paris implied in their quote above , the Kurdish musician often has a therapeutic function. The musician is the authentic transformer of emotions; she is the creative source carrying out especially the grief, pain and mourning of the individual and the society. She brings out her personal pathos and allows her environment to listen to her. She shares her burden and vehemence with neighbours, family or friends. To share her private, smarting or torturous disappointments and her sensibility, she has to dare to impart it to her environment whether or not others will understand or accept it.

Another musician from the prominent Kurdish group, the Kamkars, illustrates this fervent connection through music as follows:

> Kurdish music has the endless continuity of a stormy ocean– the hurricane of life's misery, smashing gigantic waves upon the rocky shore. Happiness, grief, work, struggle, friendship,

separation, belief and tradition all find expression in the music (Hooshang Kamkar, *Nightingale With A Broken Wing*).

Kurdish music is passionate, tremendously influential to the listener and with healing character. To structure personal hesitations and sentiments in the moment of the performance demands a creative form. To express these forms in an unpretentious way requires primary techniques. To improvise a primitive melody and sing it through the voice seems to be a secure, gratifying exercise. It is work, hard work, to individually improvise and create one's own words, melodies and forms. But I believe that this soulful transformation of sentiment and associations through authentic singing is healthy–for both singer and audience. I agree with Poché that those authentic voices have therapeutic character.

SPIRITUAL SINGING

Besides this strong profane music, tradition Kurdish culture conveys also music of religious heritage. In Sufism, the mystic tradition of Islam, music is integral to ecstatic spiritual worship.[40] Mevlana, the medieval Sufi Master, sees sickness as being cut off from everything and everybody. Healing can only come through connection and re-integration. This connection and re-integration is obtainable by everybody. Through various chanting litanies, dancing and a characteristic intense technique of breathing to pronounce the name of God, the performers lead themselves into astonishing trances. These spiritual ceremonies with religious songs are called Sama/Sema or Zikr/Zekr, depending on the language they belong to. The vocal sounds, which are often unconsciously voiced at climatic moments during spiritual gatherings, have been used for rhythmic prominence as well as for further stressing the states of trance. The singing style is an amalgamation of the contemplative with the ecstatic, requiring virtuoso performing ability, and includes the non-singers in a kind of ecstatic listening–not unlike the power of trance I described in Chapter V.

The depth and eccentric beauty of this singing style personally transported me during a concert of an Iranian Kurdish group of a mystical order.

40. Kurdish religious uniqueness has also been formed by Sufi brotherhoods with such eccentric practices as ecstatic utterances, trances, fire-eating and self-mutilation. Sufi rites are also found in other communities with 'folk' Islam and pre-Islamic religious rites and exercises. In orthodox Islamic groups Sufis were looked upon with great suspicion. In the past it was usual that different religious groups lived together. Jews have lived in Kurdistan as traders and artisans for over two millennia, as well as Christians and Armenians mostly concentrated in eastern Anatolia, and Assyrians around the Syrian hills and mountains. Kurds and Armenians possibly share the same racial roots since the last ones were established in the sixth century BC in the same area.

Seeking to revitalize the mind and promote the spirit, the Razbar ensemble presented the sacred tradition of song, chant and dance of the Kurdish Ahl-e Haqq, a mystical order dating from the 15th century[41]. Emerging out of the Sufi tradition this group preserved the deeply sacred dimension of its music. Often inaccessible for outsiders of the Ahl-e Haqq communities in Iran, the group Razbar, which resides in Germany, presents the essence of authentic mysticism combined with sociocultural changes: their purity of tradition during performance is conserved, while concessions are made by admitting women to the practical ceremony that was formerly reserved for men. Inspired by divine sources through singing chants, the Sufi practice awakens the intense spiritual feelings and emotions in every human soul. Only through heart energy and divine glory will the *zekr* bring benefits to the souls of the participants. Sharing their ceremony in public means offering something of their spiritual state, as opposed to giving a performance.

Fifteen performers, women and men in white clothes, meet in a circle on stage, symbolizing the unity of their hearts and the elimination of all social distinctions. Three instrumental players start with an introduction on tanbur (lute), Kamancheh (fiddle) and daf (frame drum), while the group attunes their bodies by gentle rhythmical movement. The group breathes rhythmically, humming and singing softly, finally forgetting the presence of the audience. One by one, each awakens through his/her own vocal utterances, prayers and calls to God, intensively chanting and moving the body. Their rigorous breathing, movements and intensified singing engage some of the performers to reach a stage of nearly violent trance. Connecting themselves with their inner personal states through the physical contact of their breath deepens their authentic vocal experience. Each individual voice sounds enormously passionate; the trance touches other singers, reaching out with profound emotional expression, evoking sublime, scary or even horrifying stages of consciousness. One observing member of the group serves to calm down the forceful singers in trance and ensures that they are under control, touching them and reorganizing their place in the circle.

Finally the whole group moves to a powerful force of collective ecstasy, a commonplace occurrence for Sufi communities. Their authentic vocal sounds include crying, internalized weeping, and severe screams of strong

---

41. Ahl-e Haqq, means 'People of Truth,' living mostly in Kurdish regions of Iran, Iraq and Turkey. The members of the Ale-e Haqq community believe that status and material possessions are of no consequence in the eye of the heavenly Beloved (Leyli, Razbar Ensemble). Ahl-e Haqq religion contains many similarities to the Alevis. Both are based on the Zoroastrian religion, founded c. 600 BC by Zoroaster also called Zarathustra. This ancient form of belief influenced Judaism, Islam and Christianity. Essential for Zoroastrian are purification rituals for the prevention of pollution, caused by spiritual, supernatural forces that arise directly from evil.

emotions. The serenity of the ambiance and extraordinary intensity of the ceremony are palpable. These individuals have moved away from being 'ordinary,' reaching sacred stages of connection with or to divine possession through fanatical continuous singing.

In my experience of the Razbar, the audience was involved in several trance-like moments. I wondered if there was a secret to its archetypal poetic imagery, melodies or singing techniques, or to the vibrant, energetic environment of the nearly frightening performance. The Razbar are people living normal lives with normal jobs in a modern society in Germany. Their energy was a mélange of relaxation and deepest devotion. I sensed the occurrence of a transformation of myself from listener into an extended spiritual unity.

When I compared these Kurdish musicians' vocal expressions, all of their voices sounded like passionate cries or screams: cries from the heart of a wounded beast, screams of souls, smashed, crushed or curled, coping with the unbearably powerful affirmation about the hurricane of life's misery. The similarity among all of them lies in the depth of sorrowful expressions through the voice. This method of improvised singing helps the person to make frank, authentic sounds. And in the Kurdish tradition of these vocal expressions, the sound of a broken soul is getting a voice, a voice connected to oneself. In these personal moments of misery, the Kurdish individual finds escape by evolving to higher degrees of order. Passionate singing and musical crying and screaming as forms of personal purification kept in order for centuries in this culture.

ISLAMIC "SINGING"

This musical and spiritual ecstasy of the Sufis is not treasured in orthodox Islam. During the Islamic periods music took on a lower role while poetry was always a higher art; in some orthodox Islamic traditions music is even totally forbidden or associated with vulgarity. Arabic and Islamic scholars and theologians were hostile to both sacred and secular music, maintaining that singing and performing were too intensely sensitive, and questioning the morale of the musicians. Considering the Sufi mystic tradition, where music is essential to ecstatic worship and passionate expression, some orthodox Islamic groups excluded Sufism from belonging to Islam. Until recently the status of Sufi music in the larger Islamic culture has been ambiguous, and the orthodox are still hostile toward it.

Another religious issue surrounding Islamic belief and doctrine involves the semantics of Koran reading practice. Orthodox Islamic groups exclude music from their traditional celebration and rituals. Reading the Koran is an integrated part of this celebration and needs musical skills, like those used in singing. After years of dispute, finally a compromise was attained in the search for an accepted practice involving the performing of the Koran. To dissociate the Koran from its musical background, the decision was made never to call it 'singing,' but 'reading' or 'reciting.' In Larousse's opinion, from the strictly musical point of view, there is no fundamental difference between the cantillation of the muezzin and the vocalizations of a professional lay singer. Sing-reading of the Koran requires a good voice, musical skills and correct intonations of the Arabic language. It never was based on a *maqam,* the structuring scale in music. But it seems that the ritual of sing-reading the Koran is the most musical daily practice in Islamic tradition today. Even though it is not considered singing, five times a day the muezzin uses his voice with micro-intervals and melodic lines to call for the celebration of God; it must have a strong effect.

As early as the ninth century an Islamic scholar, Ali al-Dunya, damned instrumental and vocal music almost completely. Others, such as Abu Hamid al-Ghazali in the twelfth century, defended it. Al-Farabi, an Islamic musician and scientist also from the ninth century, created one of the first forms of recognized music therapy, healing mind and body through the connecting power of music. He stated that the body is sick when the soul is weakened, and when the soul is sick the body is weakened. In his approach the self-healing capacity of the body gets stimulated; mind and spirit come together through the power of music, and the unity of soul and body makes healing possible. The musical scales in this approach are various and practicable for different times of the day, different personalities, and different goals. Through the various scales or *maqams* (around 400), and the subtle microtones, the virtuoso sound is applied to reach individual body parts and organs.

The Turkish music therapist and Sufi master, Güvenç, using this ancient knowledge and working with neurologists, is testing his oriental musical sounds on Western ears. He has created places in Europe to study this old oriental form of music therapy, learning to play and perform in this tradition. In Eastern as well as Western societies Güvenç's music encourages intensive listening, and when successful the listener will experience archetypical pictures of specific landscapes, animals and trance-like imaginations. These can inspire healing or stimulate accepting processes as Özelsel[42] describes them: an image

42. Michaela Özelsel, a psychotherapist in Germany educated in Middle East philosophy and Western psychotherapy, combined both. She describes the differences between the Eastern and Western approaches to thinking about life. Following her, in the Eastern thought no negative prototype of human being exists; in the Western world negative prototypes exist with the example of the sin-concept of life. In Eastern philosophy there is always hope of change, nothing is really fixed and settled down, there is always movement, as with their nomadic background.

of human beings is made in combination, for example, between angels and animals. We are not angels but we are also not animals. Both angels and animals are perfect as creations, angels are only good and animals are only following their instincts. Human beings have to learn to educate themselves and their instincts, but they should not suppress but *integrate* those parts. They will become a creature–an angel with wings and a tail of a donkey. This view means that we have to accept ourselves, both light and shadow. We have to learn to deal with both of these parts and it means allowing ourselves to resonate together in the shared world space of animals and angels.

Singing and dancing are an active part of Güvenç's therapy, which requires the client's participation and plays a significant role in waking up the body, part by part, stimulating the energy flow, and activating the body, mind and spirit, integrating all.

Orthodox Islam did not eliminate traditional forms of singing and dancing in the different Islamic cultures from the Middle East to North Africa. In the Arab world of music around the Middle East and North Africa, the storyteller or epic singer is still central and everything is done to enhance the capacities of the human voice. I already described the use of rich improvisational singing in Kurdish music, a Middle Eastern Islamic, but not Arabic, culture. A variety of traditions and different language-families are accomplished in this area.[43] And their diversity of sounds, music and tradition are gigantic.

The Arab Bedouin tribes in North Africa, for example, originally a nomadic culture, have particular song and singing traditions. As in many of the nomadic cultures, their music is regularly modelled primarily by singing with hand-clapping and feet-stamping as percussive support, combined with dancing. The *huda* are songs composed by camel-drivers with rhythms that mimic movements of the camel's feet, connecting themselves to the rhythm of their camels, imitating them and feeling empowered through them. Other songs are created for charming "against the spirits of the desert," outlining protection mainly in dry areas, or various forms of 'funeral laments' (Larousse, 1987, p. 37).

Among the Pashtun in Afghanistan, the largest ethnic group of this country in the melting pot of Central Asia, Near East and India, many individuals hide their interest in music and dance to gain religious respect. But the improvisational art of amateur singing with a concentration on poetic texts is still valued. The *landay* is a traditional song form where a nine-syllable verse is followed by a thirteen-syllable one, with words set to a rhythm. The singers habitually use a single melody to perform many *landays*. Mostly women

43. The Middle East and North Africa has a rich linguistic and ethnic variety. Different language groups stretch from the Indo-European family, with Kurdish and Persian to the Altaic family with Turkish; from Afro-Asiatic family with Semitic languages such as Arabic and Hebrew, to Berber languages of North Africa.

compose these songs in a range of types which are then performed by men. This tradition of the female composer might come from pre-Islamic times. For contemporary times it is remarkable because women normally do not play any instruments and follow their roles of being humble and not expressive as demanded by this strict conventional society. But most important, the singing culture in Islam, performed by men and women, is varied and vibrantly alive. Despite all the restrictions, authentic singing stretched through centuries, geographical distances and cultural rituals right up to today.

Chapter X

In this chapter, various connecting and healing practices from history as well as from modern surgery rooms are linked through the tradition of Native American collective singing. *Native American-Navajo Singing* identifies historical and political conditions of Navajo people and their misery, using song and ritual as an integrative process of reorganization from a personal to a communal harmony. In *Survival Singing* I portray powerful Navajo singing practice as cultural preservation and personal survival while suffering. Using the collection of *Healing Songs*, I describe Navajo collective healing rituals and the practice of finding balance between the different dimensions of life. A path to health is the concept of *hózhó*–being in harmony with Mother Earth. While sickness is seen as a result of being disconnected, the central role of the voice is to reconnect for health. *Harmonious Singing* portrays the use over the centuries of shamanic singing rituals during illness; here, Dr. Lori Arviso Alvord, a Native American surgeon, illustrates integration of songs to carry out harmony during her medical practice.

NATIVE AMERICAN–NAVAJO SINGING

While Western technology and modernization finds its peak and its limitations, I believe that there is the increasing need for serious inspection of the wisdom of indigenous peoples. My interest and travels into different cultures with authentic singing traditions has taught me that these people probably can reconnect us with ways to heal and to look at life with different, new as well as ancient perspectives steeped in wisdom traditions.

While I visited the Southwest of the U.S., I became curious about the heritage of indigenous American people, the American Indians. Respecting the strict codes of their culture–not being allowed to their ceremonies (only by invitation), no photographing or tourist trouble–I was able to watch a village ritual on my trip to the Four Corners (Arizona, New Mexico, Colorado and Utah).

Standing outside of the ritualistic circle in the burning sun in mid-August, I observed hundreds of men and women dressed and decorated with tree branches dancing barefoot in smouldering sand. The singing, dancing and drumming ceremony went on for hours with no break or interruption while the heat of the day increased; every villager was involved. Searching for a shady place, I barely survived the heat, and because of this temperature I expected that some of the singers/dancers would have a calamity. However, nobody showed any sign of tiredness, breakdowns or physical/emotional attacks. I realized that trance-like moments had taken them to a different place where the heat or fatigue was not impacting them. Fascinated by what I had experienced, I started to discover more about the American Indians, the rituals that serve their health, and their culture past and present.

With the contributions of authentic Native Americans[44] belonging to the Navajo Nation, I want to show the significance of authentic vocal sounds for collective survival, help and health. By sharing personal and professional wisdom about their culture, these examples of authentic singing show the integrative process of reorganization from a personal to a communal harmony as well as a natural, social behaviour of communities in an interpersonal process.

The importance of ancient communities such as the Native Americans in harmoniously connecting human beings with their environment through songs and rituals is gaining credence around the world. This knowledge is applied through collective singing, for example, by support groups, both in and outside of Native American culture and religious communities, to help seriously ill people sustain lower mortality. There are many other Native American traditions we can learn to value[45]. For example, giving birth vertically–not horizontally–using gravity to push effectively and so easing the process of labour, is tradition. The presence of the family during labour, combined with singing chants, creates a sense of emotional strength and support for the birth-giving mother. For Western women it is getting more common to use their favourite CD's when giving birth and have their partner with them in the delivery room. The similarity between Navajo and Western tradition in getting musical and emotional support is significant. When we open to listen to this old wisdom carefully, we might learn how to distinguish and re-integrate their knowledge into our daily work and life.

The Navajo nation is one of the Native American cultures with an intense and varied singing tradition. As symbolized in this blessing litany, Navajos are deeply attached to nature and their surroundings and preserve their connectedness through collective singing and praying:

In Beauty before me I walk
In Beauty behind me I walk
In Beauty below me I walk

---

44. Native American or American Indian, Red Indian–a member of the aboriginal race of America or any of the aboriginal North and South American stocks, usually excluding the Eskimos (Stein, 1966, *The Random Dictionary*).
45. Well-known also is the discovery of aspirin, originated from the American Indian wisdom and their profound admiration for nature, using the bark of the willow tree to cure pain.

In Beauty above me I walk
In Beauty all around me I walk
It is finished in beauty
It is finished in beauty
It is finished in beauty
It is finished in Beauty

"Beauty Way Chant," Dine Benediction
(Walking Thunder, 2001, p. 161).

The Navajos are living in the largest American Indian reservation in the United States of America. They are the second-largest tribal population of more than 500 Indian nations in the U.S. The Navajos call themselves *Dine*, meaning 'the people.' The Dine are situated in a 24,000 square miles of land, located in a reservation in the southwestern part of the United States spread over parts of Utah, Arizona and New Mexico. The Navajos have lived in this area probably since they migrated, between 500–1000 years ago, from the High Plains, the Rocky Mountains chain or the Great Basin. Following the language groups (see Chapter IV, *Linguistic Voices*), they possibly originated from the Athabaskans, coming from the Northwest of Canada and Alaska after journeying from Asia 2000 years ago. Currently there are no obvious dates for the arrival of the Navajos in the Southwest.[46] Navajo history is replete with descriptions of suffering from being treated as lesser human beings. Movies and stories tell of their horrible capture and enslavement by the Spaniards; awful massacres of Lakota men, women and children by the Seventh Cavalry; countless American occupations and re-settlements as in the 'Long Walk'; murder of their livestock by the American Government; mining of their lands without permission; being outlawed, punished and penalized by speaking their mother-tongue; being chastised and reprimanded for performing traditional ceremonies. The 'Long Walk' for example–the Anglo-American attempt in 1864 to kill, capture, imprison and then force thousands of Navajos to walk 300 miles from the reservation around Canyon de Chelly to Fort Sumner in southeastern New Mexico, ending in a massacre that left thousands dead–is just one of the horrors engraved into Navajo collective memory.

---

46. It is thought that the Pueblo Indians, who were living there before, introduced the Navajos to their successful farming system as well as to their ceremonies and rituals. Navajos adjusted to the many changes and influences of their surroundings easily. But in the sixteenth century daily existence was strongly altered through the arrival of the Spanish, bringing slavery and occupation of their territory, distressing all Native American tribes for centuries. Besides these negative effects there were also some positive influences such as introducing horses and sheep which eased their lifestyles practically.

Lori Arviso Alvord M.D (1999)[47] calls this misery 'historical grief': a grief for crimes of history that becomes your own sorrow. She compares her nation's suffering with the Black Americans, the Jews and the Tibetans who must tell their children of the murderous invasions of armies or captures and murders of their forefathers and mothers. In addition to the sores of history for the Navajos are new dilemmas of poverty, depression and alcoholism. Every generation has had to find a proper way to cope with their grief and anger about their destiny (p. 12).

SURVIVAL SINGING

One way of surviving, coping and curing this sorrow was the strength of the Navajos to collectively nurture themselves through authentic songs and ceremonies. The tradition of connecting to the land of their forefathers, and to nature itself, was necessary to endure their lives. The habit of these intense ceremonial manifestations through the powerful connections of performing rituals could bind all living beings together. 'Walking in beauty,' as the chant above symbolizes, is the way of life for Navajos: singing and keeping harmony between nature, human beings and spirits.

The prominence of women is custom in the Navajo culture, a matriarchal society where women connected and ruled the tribes. The ownership of the household is in the hands of women, and the recognition that children of belong to the mother's clan, not to the fathers, gives men after divorce no chance for custody of children. After marriage it is traditional for the husband to move in or live close to his wife's family. Women inherit a strong sense of self from their grandmothers and mothers, and are encouraged through traditional stories of being empowered by bears and other leading animals. This female strength is dramatized in many rituals where animals hold an impressive role. The connection to their power, imitating their cries, screams and sounds, as well as carrying small body parts as relics or protection, often serve important spiritual purposes.

One Navajo song, which was created during the Long Walk to maintain strength, to survive, to identify and to remember this adversity, is 'Shí Naashá,' meaning 'I am going':

---

47. The title of her fascinating personal book is: The Scalpel and the Silver Bear, The First Navajo Woman Surgeon Combines Western Medicine and Traditional Healing.

Ahala ahalágó naashá ghą.	I am going in freedom.
Shí naashá ghą, shí naashá ghą,	I am going in beauty all around me.
shí naashá lago hózhóó lá.	
Shí naashá ghą, shí naashá ghą,	I am going, I am going, in beauty;
shí naashá, ládéé hózhóó lá.	It is around me.

Motions for the song 'Shí Naashá
(Navajo music is mostly combined with movement):

Shí	Point to yourself and touch your fingers on your chest with both hands.
naashá ghą	Point outwards with your palms facing upward.
lago hózhóó lá, hee ya hee nee yá.	Clap your hands together on each beat.
ládéé hózhóó lá, hee ya hee nee yá.	Clap your hands together on each beat.
Ahala ahalágó naashá ghą.	Put your hands in front of you with your fingertips pointing towards each other, almost touching. Your palms face inward toward your chest. Move your palms in a circular motion, outward at the top and inward at the bottom. Both hands move exactly together. Move your hands through two complete cycles.

(McCullough/Help, 2001, p. 65, Appendix B)

Originating from this time of the hardship of the Long Walk, the song indicates "that you are going to survive, that you are special, and that you are going to live a long life (p. 62)." The connection to a community of suffering with voices venting numerous sounds, freeing their emotional energy of suppression, helped build a united strength. The women sang this song to uphold morale and hopes for their men during the imprisonment of the Navajos. Authentic collective singing let them trust that they would survive the hardship of the situation that was binding their lives, and very possibly contributed to that survival.

Music is integral to the Navajo world. Particularly important are the traditional songs, because until the 1970s Navajos were forbidden to speak, sing and perform in their native tongue. When children were heard speaking their native tongue in school, many forms of punishment were applied: washing their mouths out with soap, forcing them to clean the rest room with a toothbrush or to write three hundred times that they would not use their mother tongue again.

In this atmosphere of repression, traditional songs had to be learned by ear. If someone were able to do this, it would demonstrate his/her skills and suitability for continuing the traditional singing. No paper sheets for text and music lines were used; only memorization and certain movements lent a hand to learning the songs. Even though songs were learned slowly, some even appeared suddenly, for example, in dreams. When the singer woke up, he or she remembered the song and sang it over and over that whole day until it was really learned. Remembered songs and new songs were created and believed to be a gift of the Holy People[48]. Singing and dancing in a sacred way brings forth the power of the Holy People. Navajos believe that they can protect themselves, celebrate nature, warn of or fight back enemies and their environment through spiritual forms of authentic singing. Navajo treasures of songs are various and the clear differences between the functions of the song allow them to be used for specific purposes:

'Powwow[49] Songs' serve both social and spiritual desires. They represent a long tradition of community song and dance. 'Spiritual Songs' are meant for singing in the 'sweat-lodge,' a traditional sauna meant to purify body, mind and spirit. 'Ceremonial Songs' honor people, deities or nature. 'Healing

---

48. Holy People, the Gods or deities are instructors of the Navajo creation story. Their creation story is the foundation for their healing ceremonies and indeed for their entire way of life. The evolution tale of Navajo reveals the whole spectrum of their beliefs, from the physical geography of their environment to their daily behavior as dictated by the Holy People (McCullough/Help, p.27).

49. The term "powwow" originally referred to curing ceremonies. The term passed into English as a word referring to any Indian gathering or a verb meaning "to confer in council." In Indian country, it came to mean "a secular event featuring group singing and social dancing by men, woman and children." (Blumenfeld, p. 88).

Songs' are usually only sung by ceremonial practitioners, who apprentice for years, learning precise performing styles and specific song sequences. 'Sacred Songs' are directly connected to the spirits and may be sung only by certain singers in specific circumstances (Mirabel in Blumenfeld, p. 88).

HEALING SONGS

Navajo tradition has songs for everything; various songs relate to everyday activities, children's games, songs about occupation and tasks, songs about protecting animals, social songs and songs about their beloved nature, the land of their forefathers and mothers. Navajo healing songs are prominent in collective ceremonies where harmony or balance can be established or restored. The word *hózhó* in Navajo language has scores of meanings: goodness, harmony, balance, beauty, happiness, orderliness, blessedness, pleasantness, perfection, success, and well-being. This word applies to the holistic philosophy of the Navajos where "no religion is existing because everything is religious." Everything and everyone in life is connected and influences everything else: a balance between the different dimensions of life is necessary to create a path to health. Sickness is seen as a result of things falling out of balance, of losing one's way on the path of beauty, of getting disconnected. The path of health is possible through special songs, songs for healing as Dr. Alvord describes. Songs are sung by the 'singer,' a medicine person[50] who prays and sings to restore a broken connection or balance.

Through the authentic voice, rhythmic, tonal and atonal humming and singing out loud with glottal stops, and guttural resonating tones coming from a deep place inside, the singer can reach far–soothing, relieving and connecting. For centuries Navajos were able to create songs to ease birth giving or to facilitate health.

Collective singing songs indicate connection to everything: the four different directions of earth provided the representation of different parts of the day, crafting relationships to everything alive. Morning, evening, summer or winter chants, singing into trance or spiritual moments of harmony, caused rushes of individual and collective memories. Navajos were cleansing their way from daily experiences into a higher order.

Even non-Navajo war veterans with posttraumatic stress disorder are able to recover and recuperate through the effective selection of traditional

---

50. Medicine person, a shaman or *Hataalii*, is literally called "the singer" who performs the healing ceremonies.

healing songs. Mostly through passionate listening and experiencing the physical vibrations of the singing community, 'white' men can also actively participate in these holistic ceremonies. It is the passionate collective sharing in the process of identification and purification, that according to the Navajos once created the world. By entering those powers they were able re-create themselves in a state of health and wholeness. This process of active identification and imagination reaches out to nature and the symbolic world around us and might well purify human beings from trauma and suffering.

The concept of *hózhó*–being in harmony with Mother Earth, the sun, the moon, the stars, with animals and humans as well as with the Holy People–is essential to the Navajo. They sing about all these elements, imitating the bizarre sounds of all living things and building bridges through songs and ceremonies. But evil and disharmony also exist in Navajo culture as complementary components of the world balance. Even though Navajos try to prevent evil through ceremonies, disharmony, for example created through witchcraft[51] or natural elements, can also be treated by several of the scores of ceremonies.

A range of treatments is obtainable, but first a general analysis has to be made before a healing ceremony can start. If a person has a problem resulting from childhood or recently appearing symptoms or signs of illness, a consultation for a specific ceremony is essential. Before a ceremony can be performed the person/patient needs to consult a diviner, somebody who has the gift to analyse a difficulty through "stargazing, hand trembling, or listening."[52] The diviner diagnoses the problem and counsels the proper ceremony for the healing. A diviner interprets the involuntary motions of his hand; he has the gift to see or hear while in a trance-like state. He discovers the cause of the problem and determines the proper ritual for a cure and recommends a singer. From

---

51. Witchcraft is believed to be widespread among the Dine. Witches or chindi are called "skinwalkers" because they go about at night clothed in the skin of a coyote or wolf. The Dine believe that skinwalkers can turn themselves into other ceatures and cause illness or death to their enemies (Walking Thunder, p. 67).

52. Hand trembling is one of the major modes of diagnosing illness for the Dine. One becomes a hand trembler when s/he is spontaneously seized by the uncontrollable trembling and shaking of their right arm (and sometimes their whole body). This is seen as a sign that the person is possessed by the spirit of the Gila Monster. Then the ceremony must be performed so that the trembling is transformed into a manageable experience used to diagnose illnesses. Hand trembling is also used to locate lost objects, identify witches, and to find an enemy. A Dine medicine person may be a *hand-trembler* and use their hands for healing, or they may limit their practice to dispersing herbs, or to chanting or singing the sacred prayers and songs. The singers who preside over major ceremonials are called *hataali*. A ceremonial or a performance refers to a complex system of rites and ceremonies typically performed over two or ten days (Walking Thunder, p. 67).

beginning to end of the ritual the patient has to undergo a kind of hypnotic state to free up his body and mind.[53]

During the ceremony the patient is called 'the one sung over,' and the medicine man or woman, called the 'singer,' carries out the ceremony. The singer has to have an excellent memory, a capacity not unlike learning a Wagnerian opera. To memorize numerous ritual acts, hundreds of poetic lines in prayers and songs, varying in every ceremony, the singer needs to practice intensively. He apprentices for years to an experienced teacher and finally specializes in only two or three ceremonies. The singer makes his voice conform to a precise timbre, using it with special techniques determined by the circumstances. Even while memorizing poetic lines, he pays greater attention to his authentic voice production–its sounds as 'connector'–than to the words themselves. Besides being the conductor of the ritual, the singer is also the master of the ceremony–not only for the patient but for his/her family; he also directs his assistants to make sand-paintings[54] if necessary. The sand-paintings are destroyed after each ceremony because of their sacredness. He also carries a sacred medicine bundle enclosing artifacts for the ritual of healing. The singer is the central person and through the specified singing an atmosphere has to be created where all of other aspects of the ceremony work together. The voice is the connector to all dimensions and gets support for its sound through instruments such as rattles, the basket drum, and especially the water drum, used by the singer to produce the resonant heartbeat.

> Most important is the singing, usually accompanied by a rattle, led by the singer but joined by all . . . who know how. Singing accompanies nearly every act and in Navajo thought it is the one indispensable part of any ceremonial; without it there can be no cure, indeed no chantway. . . . Prayers are said at intervals and communal pollen prayers occurs at or near the close of ceremonies (McCullough/Help, p. 43).

While during the ceremony the focus is on the healing of 'the one sung over,' every ritual also has a strong social component. Exhaustively singing and dancing from one to nine days, the entire family of the 'patient' is participating

---

53. If the patient is a man, he is stripped to the breech-cloth (a female patient retains her clothes). He has a single breath-feather, taken from the shoulder of an eagle, tied to his hair. As soon as it is tied on he begins to tremble violently (or should tremble) as if under influence of a hypnotic spasm. If the patient is seized with trembling, which is usually the case, the shamans say they know the malady is caused by the gods casting a spell on the patient (Walking Thunder, p.150).
54. Sand-painting: Dine term *iikaah*, means the place where the Holy Ones "enter and go." Sand-paintings are regarded as sacred living entities (Walking Thunder, p. 127).

and involved. The family assists during the creation of the sand-paintings; they also find material and buy, prepare and serve food for the guests. Relatives also help with the expenses of the ceremony and benefit themselves from it through their personal active participation[55].The collective ceremonies turn out to be social gatherings with shared songs, prayers and blessings to restore *hózhó*. The significant place for passionate interaction for Navajos happens to be the voice. Singing, or vocal noise-making, together with a kind of monotonous drum rhythm, creates the foundation for a relaxing connection into altered states of consciousness. Believing in spiritual causes for illnesses helps Navajos in their attempts to connect themselves to spiritual power. United in altered states, reaching into their higher power are facilitated through the sound vibrations of the voice, supporting their innate healing capacity, as was explained in Chapters V and VI.

There are ceremonies and songs that can only be performed during certain times of the year. A summer ceremony cannot be carried out during the winter; a specified song is sacred and cannot be completed outside of its context, written down or performed somewhere else. Sacred stories and songs cannot be described or printed otherwise it is believed they would lose their sacredness. But several songs have had such restrictions lifted and have become well-known songs and dance patterns, performed at feast and events any time of the year. For example the 'Feather Dance Song' was taken out of the 'nightway' ceremony[56] and through oral tradition it emerged as a song and dance in a social context. The text is incredibly uncomplicated, maybe one of the reasons why it became a social song: "Sís béé dááhólíí," meaning: "It's up to the belts." The full meaning of the song translates to: "It's not up to me; it's up to the belts." Both males and females perform this dance[57]. The pentatonic melody is different from the usual focus in Navajo music on the magnetic tonic, which is called the "home base" (p. 47).

Ethno-musicologists McAllester and Mitchell describe the central role of the voice in Navajo music. Both males and females often sing with robust, nasal sounds formed through subtle ornamental alteration notes and trembles. For men the voice range is high tenor and falsetto sounds as well as low with

---

55. The gifts required for major ceremonies which consist of numerous rites and performances, often require food and animals for a feast to feed the attending community as well as money, which in the case of long chants, may be over a thousand dollars (Walking Thunder, p.138).
56. Nightway or Yeibechei ceremony: a ceremony held on the last night of a Night Chant, in which all the Gods, including Talking God, come to visit the sick person (Alvord, p. 201)
57. Nevertheless Navajo dances illustrate the prominence of its matriarchal society: the females always choose the male partners and after the dance the man has to pay the woman a symbolic amount of money for this honor. Interesting is that some men hide in their trucks when the dance starts, while others happily play with their coins in their pockets, waiting to be chosen to dance.

glottal stops (stopping the air with the glottis); women sing in a medium or low range. After an introductory formula on the tonic or bass note, the melodies rise to a fifth, octave or higher above, falling down to the tonic again at the end of every phrase. The formulas at the beginning can be repeated at the end with many phrases; this has the effect of giving song styles an extraordinary consistency and obvious identity. The scales in Navajo music differ from that of other Native American music but show similarities with Northern Athabaskan music. The stress on the triad is only found in Navajo and Apache music. Their tonal systems are heavily weighted and regularly limited to the tonic, the third, and the fifth. Rhythmical patterns are two, eighth, and quarter notes with duple and rare extra beats. Meters can change if further words are added. Only a few styles use triple meter.

The texts of Navajo songs are often brief, simple and repetitive, or imply no translatable words, only repeating 'vocables.'[58] Navajo songs are extremely rich in vocables; sometimes a whole song is made of such vocalizations and "surrounds the translatable words of the text, for example, "We yaa naa naa ei yoo'oo." Only ceremonial chants contain more complicated lines of poetry with a narrative character (McCullough/Help, p. 79-83).

Arlie Neskahi, another traditional Navajo singer, describes his own music with deep understanding while debunking old clichés:

> Native American music reflects traditions which intertwine spirituality and daily life. There are songs relating to every thing, every being and every activity, ranging from commonplace and secular to the sacred and ceremonial. Nearly all Native American music is vocal, sung alone or in choruses, usually by men. These vocals are powerfully rhythmic, often featuring shouts and even animal calls. I'm tired of reading books and seeing movies that only depict Indians drumming. One of the things that distinguishes our music is that it is not beat-driven, not rhythm-driven, it is song-driven and melody-driven. We know the proper melodies of different spirits. We are carriers of an accumulated knowledge. When I sing, I feel direct connection to hundreds of years and to all the singers who came before me. For Native Americans, the singer and the drum . . . are elemental to the connections between past, present and future, and to the ties that bind all living things. (Blumenfeld, p. 88)

---

58. These are words that are primary to the song but have no exact translations, just a structured vocal expression.

HARMONIOUS SINGING

Dr. Lori Arviso Alvord pursued western scientific methods, practiced surgery in American hospitals and experienced the influences of traditional Navajo healing songs on her own patients as well as on herself. The power of the singing voice on some of her patients astonished her. She explains that to be successful with the song the "person must let the song sink into her body, and allow it to penetrate to even the cellular level of her being. In a sense she must breathe it in." Describing the physical details of a song in terms of breath and sound she maintains that a song is more than its physical appearances; it is also made from the mind, memory, imagination, community, and from the heart. Physical or spiritual, a song never represents only one aspect of its presence. "Singing comes from that misty place where human physiology, feeling, and spirit collide" and that can be a holy or religious act or an act with great power.

The singing medicine man can draw out evil from the sick patient, a process similar to catharsis. The patient can release violating spirits or emotions through the flow of authentic vocalizations. The singer's role as an active participant in the process of healing means singing a patient to wellness and health, singing to 'human harmony.' Modern medicine is in a crisis because it has found astonishing medical interventions to combat symptoms, but has largely forgotten how to heal the causes. Healing is not a one-way relationship from the doctor to the listening patient but is it multidimensional. There is also a need for the doctor to listen to the patient and to give him/her a participating role in the process of healing. Patients want to be comforted, be acquainted and involved with what is going on in their own bodies. When the healer realizes that everything is connected, his/her actions will naturally work to decrease fear and anxiety before, during and after the intervention. This is not only relevant for the patient but also for the surgeon: a doctor in a fine mood and harmony with his/her staff will succeed more often. A human voice, a spoken word, a comforting sound can influence the healing process (see also the discussion in Chapter I about doctors' voices). Dr. Alvord experienced the negative effects and serious complications on her patients and their health when members of the health team were arguing during surgery. Disharmony during the surgery combined with the patient's anxiety before and subconsciously during the surgery, might even create life-threatening complications (see footnote [59]).

---

59. "Why is it that some doctors do an operation right but their patients die? I asked. Why do some procedures go so seriously wrong? It had to do with other things besides the procedures and instruments, besides the preconditions of patients. It had to do with stress, fear, and the problems of the surgery. After what happened with Evelyn, [one of her patients who suddenly experienced a stroke after surgery while there was no medical reason to find] it became clearer to me why there

Dr. Alvord realized the influence of harmony in her work and watched and worked on her own mood swings conscientiously. She carefully observed traditional medicine men and women who came into her hospital to comfort patients. Observing them speaking in their native tongue, touching and calming them through songs, opened Dr. Alvord's eyes and ears to the importance of harmony for health. She and her colleagues learned that patients in the hospital, when treated by a singing medicine person, had better outcomes.

> If illness could be caused by a lack of harmony, could not the same be true for wellness and the ability to heal? It made sense that if the healing environment was more "harmonious," a patient might return to wellness faster. (p. 74)

Dr. Alvord experienced regularly the power of authentic singing with some of her other patients, for example an advanced cancer patient; unexpectedly, hope appeared in the face of the man, his heart rate and blood pressure became steady and stabilized after the medicine man finished singing his song. Only if a dying patient has hope and emotional strength in combination with harmonious medicine, can a doctor aid him. The songs of the medicine man can generate this hope, creating to bridge between life and death, calling the patient back to harmony, similar to the examples of comatose patients in Chapter VI.

Empowered by her experiences Dr. Alvord has spoken at high schools, universities and at Stanford Medical School about what she has learned: to respect her patients, to empower them, and to acknowledge each member of the medical team. For treating a patient's illness everything matters: our and their efforts, their spiritual health, the health of their relationships, and their comfort and trust in the surgery, she says. Creating a harmonious relationship with her patients so they could better tolerate the operating process became possible for her through involving the patients' spirits. Her dream for a hospital with a holistic healing approach is a place with lots of light and warmth, with smells of nature, generous seating, round windows viewing the garden with colourful

---

were so many difficulties. I had operated on a patient I hardly knew, stepping in for another surgeon (something we all try to avoid) at the last minute, assuming that all would be well. I had not developed any bond of trust or acceptance in advance. During her operation, her body had been anything but cooperative, and I cringed when I thought of how either Evelyn or her spirit may have listened as I ranted during the surgery. She had no doubt sensed my discomfort, fatigue, frustration, and anger. And the nurses had argued with each other. Even when patients are anesthetized, there is some evidence that they hear what goes on during surgery and respond to what is happening. Some surgery or anesthesiologists will play music while operating. This is in part for their own enjoyment, but is also must soothe the patient." (p.74).

flowers–and a trustfully harmonious teamwork; a place where "illness as a lack of harmony" can be treated by restoring it.

Using songs to evoke harmony for healing is tradition in Navajo culture. Using harmonious songs together with established medical practice is slowly gaining credence in Western culture. We must dedicate ourselves to "[w]orking with communities, and creating bonds of trust and harmony. We must learn how to sing," Dr. Alvord concluded in her plea for the connecting power of the authentic voice (p. 16).

With this limited collection I have hoped to show the incredible diversity of the use of the voice in original forms of authentic collective singing. (For more examples, see Appendix B.) While I have attempted to address the entire scale of human expression, I am aware that this microcosm of vocal potency is necessarily incomplete. There is still so much to learn, understand, and conserve from our indigenous and traditional cultures. These examples are the reflection of the ancient and contemporary practice of community existence, problem resolution, protection and survival of a vital part of the world. The use of vocal sounds for connection with the past, present and future is not only essential for the Native Americans but it is endemic to every culture. These vocal traditions show us how to connect with spirits and nature as the source of our human existence. They also connect us to more than only individual power; they direct the purely subjective and personal towards the place of interpersonal contact and to more objective and universal experiences beyond.

Chapter XI

This chapter about conventional 'sophisticated' singing and refined singing cultures demonstrates the complexity of modernity as well as its loss of natural sound in various old and contemporary practices. In *Cultivated Singing* I discuss the Indian music practice of scales, microtones and the superior importance of voice, the most beautiful and appropriate instrument for all musical interpretations. Silvia Nakkach takes us to Ragas, Rasas and Shrutis (microtones) of Indian music while I travel through *European Singing* and demonstrate natural sounds and microtones in early forms of folk music as sung by troubadours and storytellers. In *Perfectionist Singing* I research bel canto and classical singing techniques, whereas the vibrant classical voice of perfectionism, Maria Callas, shares her fascination for the natural sounds of her singing birds. In *Western Singing,* I consider the tradition that has captured new interest in natural voices through pop, jazz and contemporary music. Perhaps rap music–with its spontaneous, speech-like form–supports Western recognition of the original beauty and importance of natural vocalizations.

CULTIVATED SINGING

I believe that the voice was in the ancient cultures and is still today over the whole world the most spontaneous way of creating authentic human sounds. Through primitive as well as cultivated expressions, the voice has extended its soverein power to the four directions. Teaching techniques for trained, technical use of the voice have become popular in many places, and the awareness of the body has entered into the process. The body as conscious support of the voice makes natural and more varied expressions possible. Actually the body is not a separate entity from the voice but in fact it is the whole instrument–the container of the voice, the speaker of the sound.

In Indian music, the voice is the most beautiful and appropriate instrument for all musical interpretations. The whole of Indian musical tradition is based on the possibilities of the voice, and singing has become a technique for attaining perfection. Indian instruments are made to support or imitate the sound of the human voice. A natural voice, with the most subtle and surprising music, expresses many ornaments, improvisations and personal interpretations of a melody. Also voices are trained to sing a 'drumming language,' expressing rhythmical sounds like drumming. These voices dialogue and alternate until they climax together. The quality of the voice is secondary and the volume also; the individual interpretation of virtuoso ornamentation of microtones of the scales is important. Silvia Nakkach studied and trained herself in Indian music and knows about the importance of the voice:

> In Indian music, the most important is tuning the voice, the instrument, and the mind to the "swaras," the natural tones, which we know as the notes of the musical scale, Sanskrit system SA, RE, GA, MA, PA, DA, NI related to European system DO, RE, MI, FA, SOL, LA, S[T]I. There are 22 microtones in the space of an octave in the Indian scale, those microtones are called: Shrutis, they are only performed by designated string[ed] instruments and the voice. It takes many years of solid practice to be able to listen to them and to identify them. The shrutis create the rich ornaments that characterize the Indian music, they constitute the main difference between the Easter[n] and the Western sound and an approach to vocal music, and they induce a kind of spiritual emotional consciousness to the experience of chanting and listening to music. I[t i]s [e]specially the awareness, the performance, and the subtle 'touch' of the shrutis that convey the different ragas and 'rasas' (Yoga of the Voice, 1999/2005. Voice and sonorous Yogic practices.
>
> www.voxmundiproject.com

Looking at the chart on the opposite page we see how much Western music is limited from lack of variations and microtones as forms of unique personal expressions. The luxury of the Indian microtones opens another way of understanding human expression; as Nakkach said they "induce a kind of spiritual emotional consciousness to the experience of chanting and listening to music." The scales, called ragas, support an enormously rich spectrum of basic melodies. There are hundreds of ragas and ten of them are basic ragas, from which other ragas are derived. Most of these basic ragas existed in original Western music too. The raga regard as "color of the mind" is the result of tonal arrangements ruled by cosmological and aesthetic laws, which connected with specific rhythm cycles (tal) that offer an almost harmonic counterpoint allowing the melody to develop through improvisations and composition patterns, Nakkach explains.

> A raga is complete when it achieves its tonal taste or 'rasa' which is another element in classical Indian music. In this

Western Notes	C		C# or D♭		D		E# or E♭	E		F		F# or G♭		G		G# or A♭		A		A# or B♭	B	
Indian Notes (*swaras*)	SA		RE♭		RE		GA♭	GA		MA		MA#		PA		DHA♭		DHA		NI♭	NI	
Indian Micro-tones (*srutis*)	1	2	3	4	5	6	7	8	9	10	11	12	13	14	15	16	17	18	19	20	21	22
Names of Microtones	(1) Tivra (2) Kumadvati (3) Manda (4) Chandovati				(5) Dayavati (6) Ranjini (7) Raktika			(8) Rudri (9) Krodhi		(10) Vajrika (11) Prasarini (12) Priti (13) Marjani				(14) Kshiti (15) Rakta (16) Sandipini (17) Alapini				(18) Madanti (19) Rohini (20) Ramya			(21) Ugra (22) Kshobini	

Source: Massey, Reginald and Jamila, *The Music of India*, Kahn and Averill, London, 1993, p. 21.

> musical system where raga, tal and rasa are combined, each musician is at once a composer, a performer, and interpreter, who knows the ascending and descending patterns of the scale from which the raga is created. This open structure allows the musician to improvise, while subtly and meaningfully developing the musical idea inherent to the raga, expanding music to extremes of unbelievable mastery and creativity. (Yoga of the voice. A brief note about the classical music of North India. www.voxmundiproject.com)

These original scales of Western and Indian music were common in the Middle Ages and before, well known as church scales or modes. Following is an outline of ragas and original Western music, highlighting similarities in tonal source, structure and original effect (Storms, p. 46):

(Ionian) : Morning Raga
Mood: serious, peaceful, lovely

BILAVAL 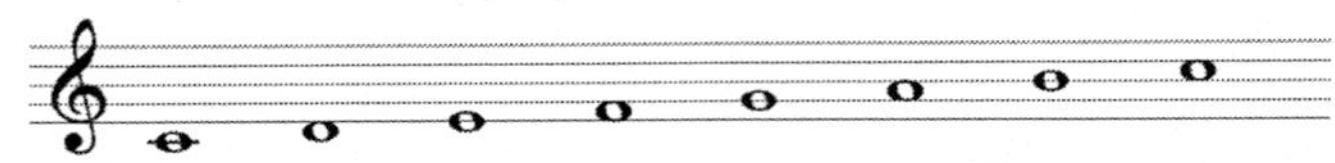

(Mixolydian) : Night Raga
Mood: longing and hope

KAMMAJ 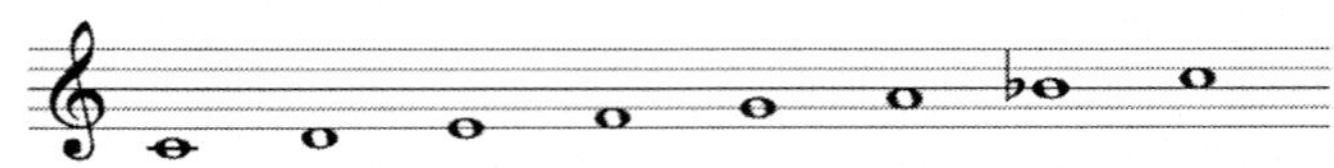

(Dorian) : Evening Raga
Mood: longing, lovely and harmonious

KAFI 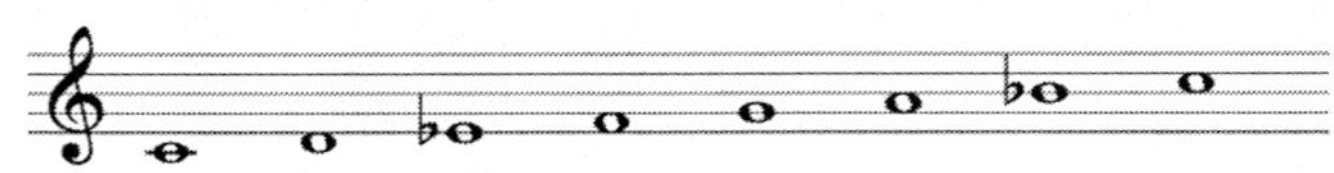

(Aeolian) : Morning Raga
Mood: melancholic; serious and dignified

ASAVARI

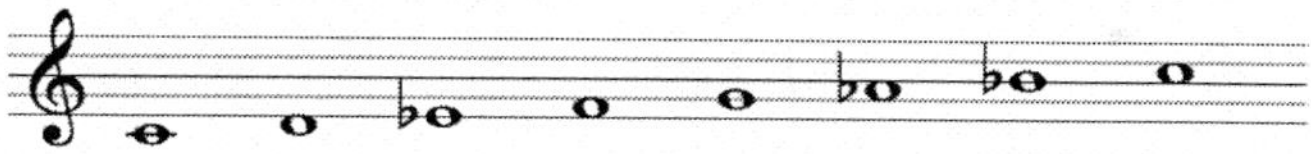

(Phrygian) : Morning Raga
Mood: sad, mixed with passion and longing

BHAIRAVI

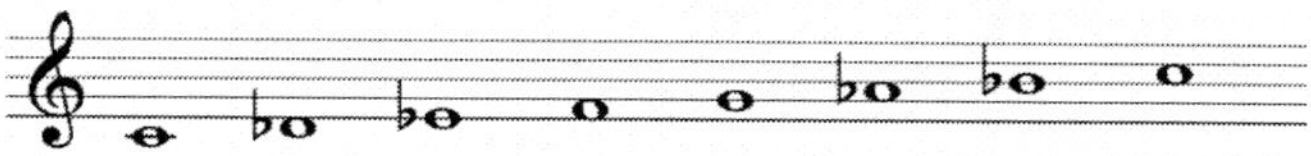

(Lydian) : Evening Raga
Mood: pleasure, with tiny melancholy

KALYAN

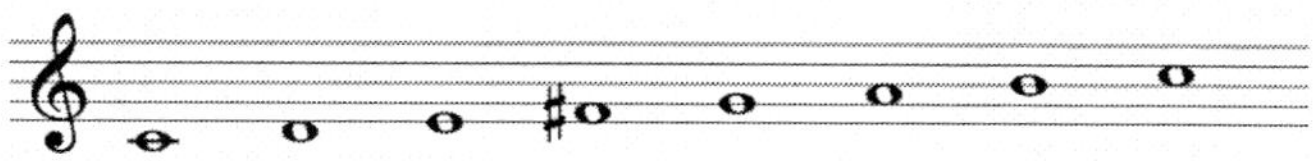

(Gypsy scale) : Morning Raga
Mood: peaceful, meditative and serious

BHAIRAV

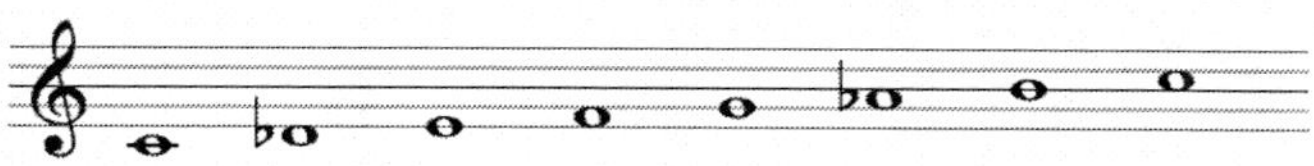

Afternoon Raga
Mood: peaceful, spiritual, serious and melancholic

SHRI

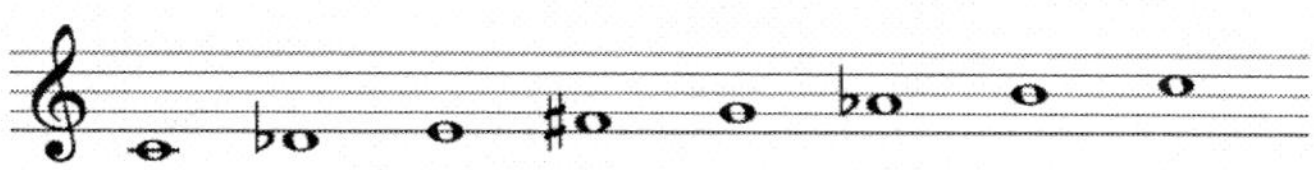

Morning Raga
Mood: serious and sad; loving

TODI

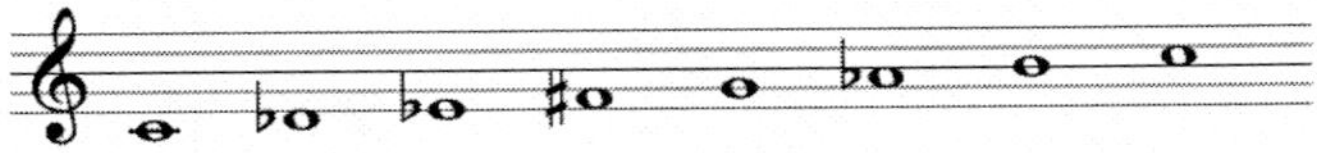

Afternoon Raga
Mood: serious, sad and unsatisfied

MARVA

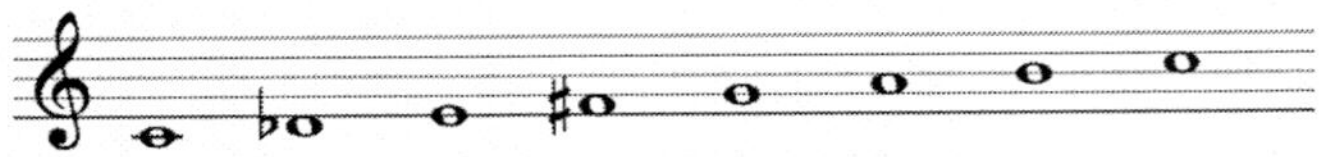

Throughout history, diversity of moods, expressing individual as well as collective emotions, seemed to frighten traditional church officials. Because of the fear about the strong impact of these musical influences, some of these ancient Eastern and Western scales became 'dangerous,' 'demonic' or otherwise not welcome, and they nearly disappeared from Western music (see European Singing). This is not unlike the dread in Islamic cultures, where music was seen as too intensely sensitive and adversely affecting the morale of the musicians. With the disappearance of various scales, a rich potential of natural musical expression was gone, including spontaneous variations with microtones, improvisations and individual, free interpretation.[60] Ritualistic and impulsive forms for conveying symbolic and unconscious messages of nature through authentic singing disappeared too.

Indian music underscores my belief that the voice is the most beautiful instrument in music. The awesome range of personal interpretation available to the singer, which allows the expression of individual colorations and nuances as an exponent for pathos, is appreciated in this and other cultures. The voice's virtuoso ability, with the paramount spectrum of human expression, active

60. Microtones can be interpreted as natural emotional vocal expressions: freeing up personal energy during improvisation in the structure of a scale, or during crying or cry-singing; in a technical sense these are small intervals; microtonality (from Greek mikro=small) is the use of intervals smaller than the usual whole-tones and semitones of the best-known Western European compositional traditions, although the use of such intervals is a routine feature of world music (see Chapter of cultivated singing.)

imagination, and direct expression of feelings and affective needs, seems to be unique in the world of musical instruments.

EUROPEAN SINGING

In early European cultures the use of the voice to express the whole spectrum of human thought and emotion was similar to the Indian form. In these times there was no notation system competent to restrict the expression of human sentiments. Vocal musical expression was a kind of experiment, dependent on the performances of priest and his singers. Through the centuries the serious chants became more complicated and often so energetic that the church authorities believed them to be unsuitable to the admiration of God. Similar to the Islamic anxiety about the power of music, in certain singing schools conducted by the church, singers were taught music theory and how to produce a tone, but were restricted in their personal vocal expression. Through this education during the Middle Ages the church became powerful in its influences:

> [The] specific demands and taboos of the church with regard to the singing voice became more conservative and stipulations demanding what could and could not be sung culminated in the infamous ruling of Pope Gregory the Great during the second half of the sixth century, whose strict stipulations led to the Gregorian chant which is still in use (Newham, 1998, p. 227).

Slowly the full, creative, spontaneous singing voice in the church tradition became more about instruction and restriction than expression. During this time, two forms of singing emerged: inside the church, with the restrictions as described above; and outside the church, still in the natural form as musical experimentation with songs of love, lust and adventure. Outside of the church the voice was still the very creative and active agent of human expression. The troubadours (or 'bards'), the European singing poets, full of passion and adventure, wandered through countries to tell their stories and tales with music. All of them kept stories, myths, mystery and indigenous religions of their culture vocally and virtuously alive. Knowledge about the songs often originally came from these indigenous traditions of singing as a healing art, with personal interpretations of variations and microtones. This tradition, as explained with many examples in the authentic singing chapters, combined the creative skill of the singer and healer in a single person.

I discovered that in possibly all of the originally primitive and later sophisticated cultures, it was normal in the oral tradition to compose poems and songs in the moment of the performance. It seems that the performance functioned also as a healing or coping strategy for dealing with feelings, imagination, and individual and social subjects. Every performance was uniquely suited to the current situation, and the bard's techniques and song construction, though sometimes influenced by others, was always his own creation.

Looking at the tradition of Lament, Kurdish and Navajo music, and the examples above, there appear the same original, common features: the personal imagination and interpretation of a song with its authentic, various forms of improvisation, colorful timbres and ornamentations. Also the European singers, the troubadours or bards, rooted in the acoustic symbols of crying, screaming, shouting or animal imitations, used the micro-intervals and sliding tones for natural expression and ornamentation. These natural tones are still audible in Indian, Kurdish, Arab, Lament, American Indian and many other music cultures. These are emotional expressions that free up energy with a healing effect.

In Central Europe, the folk singing tradition has special affective and vocal techniques, which carry these kinds of unique natural tones. Though they are all using natural sounds–acoustic symbols–the actual technical use of the voice varies from country to country:

> As we move away from the influence of the Mediterranean and the Orient, still strong among the Bulgars and the southern slaves, we shall find that vocal tones tend to become softer . . . and songs become more strictly syllabic. But although melodic melismas[61] are less frequent, the desire for ornamentation is no less strong. It makes use of other procedures, all more or less connected with the production of the voice itself, such as long-drawn-out notes opening, punctuating or closing Bulgarian songs; trill-quavers which Carpathian shepherds obtain by striking their throats with the palm of the hand; the clucking of Rumanian female singers, and the various whistles and call-and-signal cries of the mountain-dwellers of the Alps. Another specialty of the Alpine shepherds is the yodel [see Chapter IV], a technique which requires special gifts and training since it consists of the uninterrupted transition of a low or medium vocal sound system to a shrill register, or of chest- or throat-voice to a falsetto. Although the original

61. Melisma = Greek: melodic variation or coloratura.

> purpose of the yodel was long-distance communication between shepherds in the mountains, it gradually infiltrated into village music-making. (Larousse, p. 46)

These techniques are natural and varied and all of them could be called authentic as with the examples of traditional singing. I cover them here to show where the European singing tradition came from before the cultivated societies limited some of its vital vocal diversity and healing potential.

PERFECTIONIST SINGING

One of the most famous cultivated singing traditions of Western culture comes from Italy: bel canto, meaning 'beautiful song.' In this tradition, the full expression of human emotions, ornamented with colourful interpretations, is formed to a perfected technique. This tradition probably goes back to the original forms of singing in the Greek theatre with the full expression of the actor's voice. Forms of primitive singing as well as the troubadour tradition of Europe have also influenced bel canto style.

With its technique of exact notation, bel canto made a big impact on the original form of natural, improvised singing. A solo bel canto singer was able to sing an entire, wide range: tenor, baritone, soprano, and mezzo-soprano. The ability to communicate the true expression of human emotions was essential through an extensive collection of timbres. A singer could give voice from the depths of the entire spectrum of human emotions: the primal sounds as joy, grief and anger. The bel canto technique taught and represented an extension of different emotive qualities through one singer's voice. The shift from bel canto to opera was a small but significant step that had far-reaching effects. The different qualities, ranges and personalities of one voice became separated into parts or vocal categories during the development of the opera tradition. The extended expressions of human emotions through only one voice were now canalised into women and men, high and low, lyrical and dramatic sounds of voices. These specifications created separation and could afterwards effect emotional isolation. While bel canto taught human beings how to use the voice perfectly, opera taught them how to make this specification into a professional habit. The natural improvising voice that could spontaneously adapt motives, melodies and variations–the authentic way of singing–died when the opera tradition became substantial.

It is interesting to note that one of the most vibrant voices in opera, Maria Callas, was fascinated by the natural sounds of her three singing birds.

She wondered how such a tiny creature could sing all those notes, with "astonishing agility and spontaneity." Callas tried to imitate those natural sounds herself. She touched David's (her favourite bird's) throat to extort his technical secrets. Especially in times of hardship or sorrow she found comfort and company through listening and singing with them. Letting her voice naturally slide without any technical limitations, she expressed her authentic sound. Later when she was talking about her singing studies she said, "I learned more from David than from all my professors at the conservatory" (Callas in Allegri, p. 20).

WESTERN SINGING

For many centuries in Western cultures, the canalised perfectionist way of singing was the most accepted one and it influenced, and even killed, countless forms of authentic and traditional ways of singing. Of course the folk music tradition kept going and the original songs with personal improvisations survived outside of the concert halls. The natural voice was and is still used, but since opera, a voice is now often judged as ugly or beautiful, a separation that silenced many authentic singing voices and limited their healing capacity. Perhaps, in general, the individual interpretations of improvised singing, as the troubadours did, became less important and the quality of the voice became more significant. But with the emergence of jazz and pop music, the role of the voice changed this trend. Still today, the personal interpretation, the improvisation or the individual performance in these styles sets the tone; it is not the quality of the voice or the music that is important anymore but the exponent of the music. In pop music, at this moment, it is even true that an 'ugly' singing voice can be extremely popular. This means there is still a big need for some kind of personal expressions of the shadow: ugliness, nastiness, boorishness, toughness and crudeness–forms of protest against the forced, civilized constructs of politeness and conformity. The need today to express the 'little barbarian' in us (as Wilber called the suppressed parts of ourselves) and to transform them into accepted daily life seems to be overwhelming. People need this barbarian's expression also to identify themselves with others and their shadows and finally to integrate them into the personality. Of course, identification with this kind of pop music can also symbolize conformity with the oppositional or rebellious aspect of the shadow; in this case, it is not truly integrated. It is still an unconscious identification but this time on the negative side. While this music is far from beautiful, it is effective and functional for daily life and serves as one way of balancing the discord in the modern world.

A pertinent vocal example of this expression of the shadow is rap music: a long, improvised personal story about the hardship of individual or community life, sung in a recitative form with a repeated rhythmic vocal pattern, with very simple, monotone background instrumentals. The personal story in rap is significantly channelled through the way the simplistic melody supports the words and lurches from side to side between musical structures, weaving a vocal pathway.

Could we rediscover, through rap, the connection to the original use of the voice in African culture? The original vocal structure of the singing tradition of Africa was, as shown in the previous chapters, spontaneous, speech-like, and from "these inarticulate articulations slowly the music [was] born." I hesitate to call rap or pop a cultivated form of singing because it is not developed by education or training in the original way that we typically think of cultivation. And both are not really integrated but rebellious socially, vocal forms. But I find that there are still some authentic voices in today's rap and pop music: a highly developed civilization is paving a new way to an old, traditional, spontaneous form of vocal expression.

After many years of classical traditional singing, to my ears the contemporary vocal music of the concert halls has a similar maturation as pop music. In the contemporary vocal music of the 20th century, composers like Stockhausen, Schönberg, Cage, Messiaen, Berio, or composers and performers like Meredith Monk[62] and Bobby McFerrin, are challenging the current limits of the human voice. After opera, when the full expression of human emotions was canalised into voice categories, modern composers began to let the singer 'jump' over the border of singing. The singer was expected not only to beautifully perform a role but sometimes was allowed and even required to scream or sigh or imitate nature and animal sounds, or to move and dance while making natural sounds. Some of these vocal discoveries started to expand the use of the voice of trained singers, promoted the use of recorded authentic voices of foreign or primitive cultures, and integrated ritualistic forms into the vocal classical repertoire.

62. Meredith Monk's inspiration is come from a "primal source–her own body" or "the early music of Europe or the sounds of the nature" says the director of Lincoln Center Festival about her. Monk thinks about her work: "I believe that the voice was an eloquent language in itself, so I wrote wordless songs using phonemes or syllables, which I chose for their particular sound qualities or rhythm." And she described the discovering of her voice: "One day in 1965, when I was at the piano vocalizing, I realized in a flash that within the voice were limitless possibilities of color, texture, landscape, character, gender, and ways of producing sound. From that time on, I began working with my own instrument–trying to discover the voices within. I explored various resonances, ways of using the breath, lips, cheeks, and diaphragm. I also worked with the extremes of my range and quick changes from one vocal quality to another so that my voice could be a flexible conduit for the energy and impulses that began to emerge." (Stagebill, Lincoln Center Festival 2000, p.20E)

Did we ever actually lose the voice's authentic potency or was it only "hidden in the basement," as Wilber described the unintegrated voices of "archaic wishes and impulses?" The awareness of its potential and the awakening of its potency will give us back our simplest and earliest instrument for fuller self-expression in daily life, for health and for artistic performance. At this time in our society, we are in a natural process of connecting the temporal tradition–after a long time of cultivation, civilization and sometimes forced limitation of the human voice–with the indigenous traditions. It is also a natural process to integrate old and new knowledge and to re-examine the eternal truths. Just in this moment, when the transfusion of music, art, culture, religions, languages, habits and food are taking place all over the world, the voice and its traditions are also able to melt together. Again, Wilber makes me aware of this unique time in which we are living, freely traversing different cultures, theories and religions: "for the first time in history, we have access to both Freud and Buddha . . . and [they] can be integrated with the mystical or contemplative traditions, both East and West, for a more 'full spectrum'" (p. 155). In Western culture, awareness is growing about ancient cultures as treasures for new knowledge. In other cultures, the Western example of life is an idol and a direction for development. I know that these non-Western cultures are losing a lot of their originality and authenticity by imitating Western examples. Every country has to go its own way of development. Our responsibility is to protect and support these authentic treasures of the East, West, South and North and to benefit from their full spectrum of wisdom. It is more than important to keep a balance between the post-modern world of civilization and the native conservatism of primitive cultures.

Part C

SINGING PRACTICE

Kate Richards Geller and Sylka Uhlig

Chapter XII

The final chapters of this book cover the range of singing practice, experiences, thoughts and material Kate Richards Geller and I have developed over the years. Describing our workshop formula gives insight into our principles. *Singing: A Personal and Professional Need* focuses on vocal dialogue, communication and the development of awareness of acoustic symbols. *A Time to Sing* is a training forum anyone can use to explore natural sounds for exploration and expansion of pitch and expression. Central to our process is *Partner Work*, explaining personal dynamics during vocal dialogue, creating a safe environment and offering a clear structure. The *Multicultural Approach* gives further information about examples of foreign songs used and supports understanding of universal vocal potential. The *Conclusion*, *Biography* and *Discography* reference our thoughts about the therapeutic relationship, safety and importance of silence, and informs the reader about sources for further study.

SINGING: A PERSONAL AND PROFESSIONAL NEED

Throughout this book I have explored many forms of authentic voice and singing; all of these vocal human expressions have developed through the habitual practice of sound making. And it is this natural habit that I wish to protect, support and stimulate through my work in therapy, in workshops, at home, and maybe around the world, wherever it may be helpful. My favourite way to do this is to create community singing events through a three-part training that I've developed with singer-songwriter and music therapist, Kate Richards Geller. Singing together, Kate and I began discovering and transcending cultures, times and places, which was quite different from anything either of us had experienced singing alone[63]. In the process, a curiosity awoke in us about the authentic nature of our voices. After two years of partner work, realizing the effect it had on us, we opened the doors of our weekly meetings and invited others to join us singing. Combining authentic sounds with musical sensitivity and therapeutic skill, this vocal practice has benefits that are both personal and professional. We offer the workshop, "Singing: A Personal and

---

63. A meeting of voices occurred in January 1999, very literally, when a group of people was instructed to close their eyes, sings one tone, and walk around the room until they found a partner voice. It might be a unison tone or a harmony. We would know it when we found it–and both voices had to be in agreement about the partnership. And so it was that Sylka Uhlig and Kate Richards Geller would begin their vocal partnership . . . eyes closed, listening, exploring, discovering.

Professional Need," in full or in segments, in NYC and at music therapy conferences, institutions and universities in the USA and Europe (see www.TouchingVoices.com).

Despite its obvious importance, the attainment of vocal skill and freedom is considered intimidating by many professionals, and thus avoided. Observing the use of the voice in music therapy at the presentations of the World Congress of Music Therapy (Washington, DC, 1999), we identified a need to develop a regular practice so that singing becomes as natural and easy as playing the piano or guitar or drum. The value of our work lies in stepping beyond the intellectual understanding of the skill and into the experience of being in the music with one's whole self. The purpose of the training is to emphasize that the most effective use of the voice in music therapy is not singing songs to or with people–it is communicating with human beings through sound. Our approach focuses on dialogue, communication, and the acoustic symbols that are inherent in authentic human sounds. The training goal is that participants will develop the skill and freedom to use the body and voice in improvisation and finally to communicate with the client. We divided the focus of our training into the following three parts, described in more detail below and elaborated in the sections that follow.

A Time to Sing focuses on the natural sounds of the voice for exploration and expansion of pitch and emotional expression. The object is to expand the range of the voice and to vocalize from the body and the imagination. Body warm-ups, vocal exercises, and listening training prepare participants/therapists to work creatively with their own natural sounds, as well as their clients'. We address important therapy issues of creating a safe space, establishing rapport and dealing with issues of intimacy. This method, which is also offered as a separate workshop for singers and non-singers, emerged from our weekly improvisations and is designed for all to experience their own voices at their own pace in a contained and non-threatening environment. The goals are process-oriented, not performance-based or goal-oriented.

Partner work involves a series of exercises interacting vocally with peers to develop versatility in hearing acoustic symbols and creating a dialogue that is meaningful. The personal dynamics that emerge in this work enhance our ability to dialogue with our clients. Clinical examples are used to support and clarify the use of the dialoguing voice in a therapy setting. These exercises were developed from our improvisations and their impact on our relationships, moving from unison into harmony and to the tonality of maternal and paternal roles during moments of countertransference.

Multicultural approach exposes us to human sounds and musical motifs of other cultures that are primitive and often universal. Listening to singing from different parts of the world, we being to understand the many sounds human beings can make and the symbolic messages they convey. We then interact with these sounds and centric melodies, incorporate them into our own repertoire of vocal sounds, and become ready to use them in therapy. The significance of these multi-cultural influences emerged from our singing together, transcending cultures, time and places, and from the extended understanding of foreign music and its connotation.

A TIME TO SING

This title of the workshop alludes to this passage in the bible: "to every thing there is a season, and a time to every purpose under the heaven."[64] The following quote also speaks to how natural singing is and how important it is to make time to do it.

> Singing is the true mother tongue of all human beings, for it is the most natural and simplest way in which we are there undividedly and can open up our hearts–together with all our experiences, our emotions, our hopes.[65]

Essentially, "A Time to Sing"[66] is designed as a weekly voice workshop, like a voice lab, that emphasizes the importance of making time for ourselves just to sing, individually and collectively. By so doing we nurture ourselves and each other and develop a practice of caring for ourselves and engaging in something that used to be so natural for us as children and is still commonplace in different cultures: singing just to sing. A simple structure of exercises is offered in the same sequence each week in which participants can experience their bodies and voices as their primary instrument, explore tonality and natural sounds, and create personal melodies within a supportive community. The most remarkable outcome we discovered was that, even though

64. Ecclesiastes 3, King James Bible
65. Lord Yehudi Menuhin, Il canto del mondo, Düsseldorf, Germany.
66. In April 1999, Kate founded "A Time to Sing" as a sacred (meaning: designated, private, intentional) space to dwell in vocal tones, explore intervals, and create personal melodies; a time to sing for yourself and with others, a time to explore and expand your vocal range (in terms of pitch and personal expression), a time to enjoy making sound without the pressure of performance or production. Sylka arrived in New York in September 1999; the program evolved into a focused collaboration of two voices exploring the boundaries of time and space and relationship. Primarily using improvisation, we, Kate and Sylka, sang together almost every week for two years. A pattern emerged from our free improvisations which became the format for the workshop that was opened up to the public in October of 2001.

the structure remained the same, the musical content of the workshop was completely different each time. Some weeks we had the exact same people and still each session was totally different. People came from different backgrounds–acting, singing, music therapy, dance therapy, finance, architecture, education–and still found something meaningful in having a space in which to sing without being judged, to explore sounds that were perhaps "not beautiful," and to express feelings and concepts that often surprised them. Consistently, participants reported feeling "better" after singing in this way.

We did not require regular attendance from participants, yet those who did attend regularly reported a benefit from the therapeutic relationship that developed through this group singing experience. As they became more adventurous in their vocal explorations, we continued to acknowledge and accept their participation by verbally reflecting our observations at the end of the group.

Using a unique model of co-leading, workshop participants engage in vocal interplay and dialogue, establishing an environment conducive to creative expression. Participants have reported feeling less intimidated when they could choose which leader they wanted to follow or remain silent or sing softly, in the supportive presence of other voices. The "Time to Sing" workshop contains the following elements:

GREETING RITUAL. Be aware of your own comfort level regarding eye contact and personal space. Notice the comfort level of group members as you greet them and respect different levels of intimacy.

- Begin singing "hello," not talking, using different vocal improvisations
- Sing with the co-leader if you have one
- Sing to the group as a whole
- Sing to each member individually
- Allow the natural development of groove
- Establish a rhythm with your feet, if needed; singing a bass ostinato in a rhythmic, repetitive pattern is essential to maintain the groove
- Move your body in the rhythm; develop a swaying pattern as with work songs, if needed
- Listen for and emphasize archetypal song forms and vocal sounds
- Groove until it ends naturally; allow yourself to be surprised

WARM-UP. Use tone internally and touch externally to tune up the body/instrument. Move from head to toe with a gentle massage, one region at a time. Massage each region with your fingertips and try to feel the vibration of your voice there. Explore your own sounds, yawns, sighs, grunts; let any natural sounds flow.[67]

Head: make sound that vibrates on the very top of your head, very high squeal or an "Ee"
Face: make sound like "Ng" or "Mm"
Throat and neck: massage with easy rotations of your neck, look to the right and left, half-yawn sounds
Shoulders: massage and tap, rub down your arms, pat them
Chest: front and back; notice your rib cage open and close with each breath, sigh "Ah"
Belly: move hips in every possible direction; sing "Oh" or "Oo"
Legs and feet: rub down your legs and pat them, stomp on the ground
Hang over like a rag doll; let sound flow on your breath–sing glissandi
Bend your knees slightly and slowly roll up, voice any natural sounds
Stand upright, open chest, gently shake and bounce and wiggle, making natural sounds
Be still and silent for a moment: feel the effects of this warm-up

LONG TONES._Open your awareness to other voices in the room while staying in the sensation of the vibration of the tones in your own body. Your individual experience is valuable information about you and your relationship to your voice.

- Exhale a tone out of silence; 'in tune' or 'out of tune'; feel but don't 'produce' the tone
- Open your senses to hear tones and perceive vibration; hear your own voice
- Allow shifts in emotional flow of energy, meet the other voices in the space between
- Allow it to end naturally, finish with sigh

---

67. For longer workshops the following sequence can be added at the end of the warm-up and repeated after the break: Stretch high to the ceiling. Lean forward and hang down like a rag doll. Cup your hands as if you are drinking water from a river. Slowly roll back up to standing. Stomp your feet on the ground to steady yourself, imagine sending roots from the bottom of your feet deep into the earth. Wiggle and bounce.

DRONE–NATURAL SOUNDS. Drone is the bass, bordune[68], ground or "one" in the scale, the center or home tone. A range of A-flat to D-flat below middle C has been useful for a mixed group of male and female voices. Allow a silence at the completion of each segment.

- Group holds the drone for the entire segment
  - Find a comfortable way to sustain drone by exploring breath, volume and body posture
  - Breathing is staggered, drone is continuous
  - Accordion, harmonium or shruti box can support drone and maintain pitch
- Take turns while group holds drone
  - Explore "natural sounds" that exist in the voice: throat clearing, whining, crying, howling, hissing
  - Search for tone before any correction is made; allow sound to emit rather than to force it
  - Explore unclear and not beautiful sounds or the opposite, all are acceptable
- Finish turn and return to holding drone
  - Returning to drone, next person takes turn
  - Offer a visual cue to neighbor, such as a nod

DRONE–PERSONAL MELODY

- Group holds the drone for the entire segment; same as above
- Take turns while group holds drone
  - Explore personal melody created out of natural sounds
  - Give melody a beginning, a middle and an end
  - Allow sound to emerge naturally from the body rather than compose melody in the mind, image what your voice wants to express[69]
- Finishing turn and return to holding drone; same as above

PERSONAL MELODY–VOCAL OSTINATO. Repeat a two-tone pattern, an ostinato, which provides a very specific experience of vocal holding: try more than one interval combination.

- Group sings repetitive pattern of ostinato for the entire segment
- Take turns while group sings ostinato pattern

---

68. Bordune: a continuing bass tone, which is heard in instruments like bagpipe or some stringed instruments; also sung through a voice.
69. See also Mitchell L. Gaynor. M.D. using the term "life song," p. 124-125.

    - Explore personal melody: beginning, middle, end within ostinato
    - Allow sound to emerge naturally from the body rather than compose melody in the mind; image what your voice wants to express within ostinato
- Finishing turn and return to ostinato; same as above

PERSONAL MELODY–RHYTHMIC OSTINATO. Add a strong rhythmic pattern which is important for orienting group to a sense of time, space and preparation to end the workshop:

- Group sings established rhythmic pattern
- Take turns while group sings this rhythmic pattern
    - Explore personal melody within this rhythmic pattern; same as above
- Finish turn and return to rhythmic pattern; same as above

ENDING. Use a song that is simple and easily learned by singers and non-singers. Spirituals or chants are ideal, for example, "You've Gotta Sing, When Your Spirit Says Sing." Begin by singing it simply, and as the group becomes comfortable with it, improvise harmonies and rhythmic patterns; allow the song to find a natural ending.

OBSERVATIONS AND SUGGESTIONS. We discovered some simple guidelines to conducting the sessions. Begin singing rather than talking. This creates an environment of mutual welcome and community. Everyone enters at his/her own rate of comfort and finds a way to become part of the group experience. We often find ourselves singing and moving in a big circle, often running or skipping at some point. There is usually a period of silliness and laughter that looks and sounds as if we are children in a playground. Sometimes there is subgrouping or pairing but that is the exception not the rule. The greeting moves through many stylistic, cultural, and dynamic musical forms before finding a natural, not forced or conducted, ending. This experience establishes a sense of group musicality–somehow everyone hears when the greeting is over without really knowing how.

After that "surprise" ending, a silence ensues which can be very interesting. This allows members to acknowledge, in a private way, what their experience was and at the same time acknowledge their presence in the group. From this moment, we find it useful not to talk but to go directly into a warm-up. If directions are necessary, they can be sung. Otherwise body language will suffice as long as it is very obvious and directed to each individual, especially those who have never done this sort of exercise. If you are co-leading, one person leads the warm-up so that the directions are clear.

Another silence after the warm-up allows time for members to evaluate their personal experience within the group, moving into the more subtle level of the long tones. Those tones can be experienced in an organic way if they are modelled rather than verbally explained. Some members are unsure of what to do initially but they catch on quickly by watching the leaders. One leader can always keep an eye open to nod to questioning looks. As in the greeting ritual, this exercise ends by itself often when the members hear a cadence or intuitively sense an ending.

PARTNER WORK

Use of the voice is an essential tool in establishing the safe and conducive space for the client to explore his/her issues. Speaking or singing, our voices are usually the very first means of contact we have with clients. The messages we convey vocally, consciously or unconsciously, are the first impressions that set the tone of the session. This structure was designed out of improvised duet singing over the course of three years on a weekly basis. We reviewed very specific patterns that we always used to begin an improvisation and created the teaching model from this. Some of the exercises are variations from vocal workshops we have attended over many years and realize there are certain basic vocal holding and exploration techniques, like archetypes, across many types of teaching methods. Other exercises are distinguished clinical forms, as written about in Part A of the book, such as the comforting singing voice of a music therapist. Seriously ill clients may connect into intimacy or altered states of consciousness through using breath, acoustic symbols and singing with or without vibrato as in coma condition. With the archetype of the lullaby, a mother soothes her child by incorporating the sounds, tonality and emotional message of the child into her song. With the natural cry or scream, a human can be comforted; "when one naked human howl meets another, the walls are gone." As explained in Part A, we believe here is the entrée to a real therapeutic relationship.

During partner work workshops we offer suggestions for exercises, explain about clinical examples, and encourage people to communicate with their own authentic sounds. Participants always are invited to follow their own needs and do only what feels right for them. An important rule is to stay with yourself and focus on your voice in your body in order to learn to listen and to connect. The workshop format is as follows:

GREETING RITUAL: Same as in "A Time To Sing."
WARM-UP: Same as above.
LONG-TONES: Same as above
DUETS. The emphasis with duets is on listening to the self and the other at the same time. When one feels lost, the goal is to turn the attention to his/her own voice and from this place of an established self, open to the other. This can be achieved without interrupting the exercise. It will be a constant practice of coming back to the self in order to really hear both voices.

- One holds drone
    - Other explores natural sounds; same as above, (after one minute, switch)
- One holds the drone
    - Other creates personal melody; same as above, (after one minute, switch)
- One sings ostinato
    - Other creates personal melody within ostinato; same as above, (after one minute, switch)
- One creates personal melody
    - Other repeats last sounds of partner's melody, then creates own melody (after one minute, switch)
    - Same but no time limit (partners determine switch)
- One imitates vocal client examples; natural sounds like cry, scream or sounds of clients heard before
    - Other creates drone or ostinato, incorporating sounds of other (no time limit–switch at will)

ENDING: Same as above

MULTICULTURAL APPROACH

The multicultural approach includes examples of foreign songs with exciting vocal sounds, helping us to understand that the use of the voice has incredible potential to express, to relax, to lament, to meditate, to imitate, to recite and to transform human emotions. The following examples are a mixture of subjects with common or out of the ordinary vocal sounds. We listen to the songs, analyse their specialty and later imitate or interact with them to practice with our vocal ability and range, and understand the meaning and feeling. One way to do this is in a step-by-step order:

- relaxed listening–opening ears, mind and body for unusual sounds
- slowly breathing–with the rhythm of the singer adjusting inhale and exhale to music
- humming–softly and tenderly internalizing and imitating the sound
- singing nonverbally–following the melodic or rhythmic line, imitating vocal sound
- singing fully–using original as example to create own personal or second melody

The following CD examples–especially *Global Voices* or any other collection of world music–can be used. With this step-by-step instruction, listening, imitating or interacting with different styles, we learn to expand our vocal range, our listening capacity, and our understanding of humankind.

World Music Examples

Example of a centric melody, rich vocal improvisational harmonic style:
1) Italy: Traditional tenors from Sardinia.
Tenores de Oniferi. (1998). *Serenada De Ierru.* Global Voices [3 CD's]: Traditional, Sacred, Contemporary. Music of the World, MOW 149. Cradle of European civilization with ancient, nearly unchanged musical tradition.
Cantu a tenores are sung to accompany the performers or singers of improvised poetry. Its polyphonic arrangement provides rich harmonics and unusual harmonies. Two guttural voices, one in tonic, one in fifth, a third voice sings the third and the solo voice sings melody. Minimalistic with repetitive micro-phrases, lyrics often improvised or inspired by poems.

Example of monotonous, meditative natural sounds, airy open tones, create trance stages:
2) **Tibet: Sacred music of monks**. Ganden Monastery Monks. (1990). *Kabsumpa* (The Three Occations, Tribute to Buddha by Tsongkhapa). Global Voices [3 CD's]: Traditional, Sacred, Contemporary. Music of the World, MOW 149.
Overtones or harmonics of human voice sung by group of men, singing one note unison, producing sound similar to several intervals. Kabsumpa is a prayer of the great Tibetan Buddhist teacher Tsongkhapa. Several monks skip their voices to signal transitions in the chant. Final note before moments of silence often

hook downward in pitch; also moments were singers spiral upward in pitch, allowing the sound to get softer until its disappears completely into air.

Example of work song (not love song), with the function of relaxing and calming animals:
3) **Columbia: Traditional music of cowboys**. Maria Olga Piñeros. (1992). *Copla De Ordeño.* Global Voices [3 CD's]: Traditional, Sacred, Contemporary. Music of the World, MOW 149.
Work song typical for cowboys from the Columbian plains to calm their cattle during milking and transport. Text is surrealistic and sings about Venus, rain clouds, butterflies and several references to Virgin Mary.

Example of natural, particular vocal sound used in a lullaby to soothe a child:
4) **Native American**: **Lullabies**. Salish (Lillooet) (Flora Wallace, Joyce Fossella, Freda Wallace). (1998). *Tzo'Kam.* Under the Green Corn Moon, Native American Lullabies CD. Silver Wave Records. SD916.
This song simply says "sleep little boy, sleep little girl" followed by a sound made by Flora with the tongue used by the Salish people to soothe a child.

Example of simple melody with hypnotic effect and microtones:
5) **Jemen**: **Traditional Jewish songs**. Ora Sittner. (1995). *Qyria Yefefia*. Global Voices [3 CD's]: Traditional, Sacred, Contemporary. Music of the World, MOW 149.
Old Jewish melody from Yemen with simple linear structure, creating a hypnotic result. Ancient Hebrew poetry; melody is traditional song from later times. Much of Hebrew-Yemeni music served as a model for later music of Israel.

Example of lament, strong emotional quality through microtones:
6) **Greece**: **Mediterranean Songs**. Savina Yannatou and the Primavera en Salonico emsemble. (1998). *ΠΑΤΙ ΠΟΥΛΙ ΔΕΝ ΚΕΛΑΗΔΕΙΣ- Why little bird do you not sing*. Songs of the Mediterranean. CD. LYRA General Publishing Company S.A. Lyra, Greece. ML 4900.
Thracian lament for the fall of Constantinople, with the melismata and the demanding skill requirements typical in songs of this kind.

Example of meditative, repetitive airy sound, used to create trance stages:
7) **Turkey**: **Musical Sufi tradition**. Güvenç, O. and Tümata. (1995).*Veysel Qarani*. Ocean of Remembrance, Sufi Improvisations and Zhikrs. [CD]. INTERWORLD CD-915.

Zhikr literally means remembrance or recitation of God's name. Sufi practice of Brotherhood/Sisterhood produces certain states of consciousness, strengthening feelings of love, friendship, solidarity and humanity within the community through repetition of phrases of the zhikr and classical improvisations of the ney flute.

Example of improvised singing, guttural sounds, rich emotional quality in voice:
8) **Iraq: Kurdish chants**. Said Hassan. (1974). *Lo Delal Sherin Hayat*. CD. UNESCO COLLECTION 1974-1989, AUVIDIS, D8023.
This song is a typical example of Mesopotamian style, with its guttural accents, sung by the Iraqi Kurds in Kurmanchi dialect. The song is arranged around simple tones but with many vocal improvisations with micro-intervals, expressing his personal feelings. The bard (singing poet) tells the story a young man who has a dream about a woman, whom he then meets one morning. Traditionally the bard will sing and improvise until his listener is ready to depart in a soothed and relaxed mood–a kind of social therapy.

Example of breathy, nasal sound, imitation of characters in voice:
9) **Ethiopia: Traditional poet-musician**. Seleshe Damessae. (1994). *Endiawes*. Global Voices [3 CD's]: Traditional, Sacred, Contemporary. Music of the World, MOW 149.
Azmaris, a poet-musician sings in Amharic, the language of Ethopia. He sings songs of passion, sensual love, hope and social commentary. The vocal style includes a wide variety of breathy and nasal sounds. Typical for this song is that the vocal styles of the characters portrayed are imitated.

Example of warm-up sung before a ceremony starts:
10) **Morocco: Traditional Gnawa music**. Hassan Hakmoun. (1995). *Sala Alla Alik' Dima Dima*. The Fire Within, Gnawa Music of Morocco. CD. Music of the World CDT-135.
Where Arabs and Berbers meet sub-Saharan Africans, the Gnawa ceremonies are most visible. Gnawa were held to placate spirits that have inhabited a certain person or place. The musicians warm up for the ceremony with entertainment music using the three stringed lute. The drums and castanets announce to both the neighbours and spirits that the ceremony is about to begin. The clear balanced pentatonic melody and propulsive drive of the syncopated rhythms have elements from West Africa.

Example of imitation of animal sounds, fast call and response:

11) **Bali: Music Drama**. Kecac Ganda Sari Singers and Dancers. (1990). *Kecak Music Drama Interlude*. Global Voices [3 CD's]: Traditional, Sacred, Contemporary. Music of the World, MOW 149.
The remarkable vocal section of a large group of singers who precisely perform sung and spoken phrases in rapid succession; chanting "cak, cak, cak" in alteration, imitating the sounds of monkeys. The voices of officials signal the change in rhythm with their calls.

Example of recitation, bizarre vocal call and response:
12) **China: Buddhistic reading ceremony**. Dongjing music, reading of Du Biaowen (Buddhist Memorial). CD. PAN Records 2058CD, Ethnic Series.
These readings inform the gods of the participant's requests during the Donjing ceremony. The manner of reading varies from individual to individual. After the reading the instrumental music starts and the memorial is prepared for burning.

CONCLUSION

This chapter creates an opportunity to develop your own voice so as to enhance its efficacy in therapeutic and educational settings. Allowing oneself to explore all the sounds that are possible offers a freedom of range and expression that is essential in therapy and teaching. Individuals, both singers and non-singers, come to this method with a variety of fears and expectations. Many participants say that they have never sung one note–the drone–for so long. Many say they were never allowed to use their voices so freely to make natural sounds.

This intimate social experience can lead to a deeper understanding of oneself. Knowledge of the voice is the key to its impact. Regardless of our comfort level, we use our voice in every session (or class). It is our primary instrument, inseparable from our body-mind system and therefore a link to our thoughts and emotions. The more we learn about our own vocal instrument, the more responsibly and effectively we will be able to use it.

Music therapy. "A Time to Sing" was often therapeutic for participants but it was not a music therapy group. The fact that we are music therapists was significant in the creation and containment of the group experience. We define music therapy as the intentional use of the therapeutic relationship and the elements of music to effect change–physically, psychologically, cognitively, emotionally, socially, and spiritually. Therapeutic relationship necessitates establishing and developing/maintaining rapport and a meaningful, trusting relationship in which the client(s) can feel safe enough to address therapy goals. Though we are always aware of these elements in the sessions, the format of "A Time to Sing" did not require the level of commitment that would establish trust in the group; nor did it provide a space for a level of verbal processing that would take the experience to a deeper level.

Safety. Creating a safe space, or a 'conducive environment,' requires some of the following elements: consistency, communication, boundaries, compassion, and care. Establishing and maintaining a 'non-threatening environment' demands constant awareness. Singing, giving voice to aspects of oneself, elicits highly charged emotions in most people we've encountered. There is often some degree of trauma related to the voice and we have found it essential to be prepared to openly accept whatever a participant experiences. Key elements of 'safety' include clearly stated directions and expectations, consistency of environment (actual location, same structure, and/or therapeutic presence of leaders), invitation to do only what is comfortable, unconditional acceptance of participation, and eye contact.

Silence. Silence is an amazing tool for developing listening skills in this work. It becomes more valuable for regular members as they begin to notice changes in their bodies and minds from week to week. Over time an acceptance of the silent times develops and people become more comfortable with it. We create a space for silence after every segment of the workshop. One way to judge the amount of time for silence is to watch the participants for their level of internal processing versus awareness of the group and take one more breath after you feel it's time to continue.

BIBLIOGRAPHY & DISCOGRAPHY OF MUSIC OF NATIVE CULTURES

Similar to the CD examples pertaining to the voice, following is a list of books about the specific use of voice and music from multicultural perspective. These suggestions reflect our recommendations, and represent some of the sources from which we developed our techniques and methods. The discography at the end completes the treasure of world music in general with some non-vocal selections.

Alvord, Arviso Lori, M.D. & Cohen van Pelt, Elizabeth (2000). *The scalpel and the silver bear: the first Navajo woman surgeon combines western medicine and traditional healing*. New York, Toronto, London, Sydney, Auckland: Bantam Books, Random House.

Blumenfeld L. (Ed.)(1993). Book and CD's. *Voices of forgotten worlds: Traditional music of in indigenous people.* Roslyn, New York: ellipsis arts… Produced in Cooperation with the United Nations Centre For Human Rights.

Cook, P. M. (1997). Book and CD. *Shaman, Jhankri & Nele, Music healers of indigenous cultures.* New York: Ellipsis Art.

Holst-Warhaft, G. (1992). *Dangerous voices, women's laments and Greek literature.* London and New York: Routledge.

Karolyi, O. (1998). *Traditional African & Oriental music.* Harmondsworth, Middlesex, England: Penguin books.

McCullough-Brabson, Ellen & Help, Marilyn. (2001). *We'll be in your mountains, we'll be in your songs, a Navajo woman sings.* University of New Mexico Press.

Khan, Hazrat Inayat. (1983). *The Music of life.* New Lebanon, NY: Omega Publications.

Bradford Keeney, Ph.D. (Ed.) (2001). *Walking thunder: Dine medicine woman, profiles of healing.* Philadelphia: Ringing Rocks Press.

Discography of World Music

Shajarian Alizadeh Kalhor. Masters of Persian Music; *Without you.* CD. World Village 468011, harmonia mundi.

Yuri Yunakov Ensemble. *New Colors in Bulgarian Wedding Music.* Traditional Crossroads CD 4283, (1997).

Kayhan Kalhor & Shujaat Husain Khan. *Ghazal, Persian & Indian improvisations.* CD Shanachie 66011.

Radio Tarifa. *Rumba Argelina* and *Temporal.* CD World Circuit/Nonesuch 79472-2 and 79499-2.

Paul Winter Productions. *Living music*. Earth Music Production, LMUS.

Djivan Gasparyan. *Moon shines at night.* CAROL 6604-2, GYROSCOPE (1993), CD All Saints Records LTD.

Glen Valez. *Breathing Rhythms* and *Seven Rhythms for Toning* and *Revitalizing the Chakras.* CD's. Sounds true, STA MM00120D and M006D. CD's of collection of frame drums with overtone singing. ellipsis arts…

Voices of Forgotten Worlds. *Traditional music of indigenous people.* ellipsis arts…

ellipsis arts… *Celtic, pygmy, experimental, celebration, pan-African…* productions, 1-800-788-6670, 6670; elliarts@aol.com

Native American Lullabies. *Under the green corn moon.* CD. **Silver Wave Records,** SD 916.

Putumayo World Music. *Music of the whole world.* CD. One World, PUTU126-2.

Global Voices. *Traditional, sacred, contemporary.* 3-CD set. Music of the World, MOW 149.

Bobby McFerrin. *The Voice.* (and other CD's) CD. Elektra/Musician 960366-2.

Mariza. *Fado Curvo.* (and other CD's) CD. Time Squares Records. TSR-CD-9033.

Jonathan Hart Makwaia. *the wild is rising*. CD. Jonathan Hart Makwaia (ASCAP) 2000 JHM 1299.

Montserrat Figueras. *La Voix de L'emotion The Voice of Emotion.* CD. Fontalis ES 9901.

Rhiannon. *Rhiannon's interactive guide to vocal improvisation.* CD. Sounds True.

Traditional Buddhist Music from Tibet, China, Korea, Ski Lanka and Japan. *One Sound.* CD 4015, 2000 ellipsis arts…

Le Mystere des Voix Bulgares. CD. Elekra/Nonesuch. 979201-2.

Madredeus. *Ainda*. CD. Metro Blue. CDP 7243 8 32636 2 2.

World lullabies sung in Native Voices. *The World sings Good Night*. 2 CD's. Silver Wave. SD 803 and 909.

REPRISE

People all over the world express themselves primarily through their voices–crying as baby, screaming as infant, shouting, laughing, talking or singing about the sun and the moon, nature, relationships, neighbours. Mothers sing to their children to make them feel safe and relaxed; lovers sing to each other to depict their love; friends sing to share pleasure and sorrow; therapists sing to contact and comfort their clients; relatives sing to express happiness and grief; communities sing to survive and connect; children sing for themselves to discover the world. . . . Humans sing.

The acoustic symbols of 'vital consciousness' are waiting to be awakened so we can reclaim the primitive, authentic voice as a healthy instrument for contact and communication between all human beings. The simplicity of the melodies of primitive music and vocal expressions of infants, the property of their repetitions and natural relaxing effects, are significant material for therapeutic use. Through the paramount spectrum of human expression, active imagination, and direct expression of feelings and affective needs, spontaneous vocalization supports the movement from chaos to order, individually and collectively. It is important to realize that the vocal and sometimes ritualistic connection is more than individual power; it is what transmutes the purely subjective experience into the objective, and this movement can overcome serious isolation.

In today's industrialized, civilized cultures, in this highly technological society with many restrictions imposed on the use of the voice, is it important to urge people to realize the wonders, truths and effects lying dormant in their voices. Recovering from its limitations and slowly reclaiming a more natural, authentic sound, rediscovering and re-experiencing the range and potency of the voice, including the shadow sounds, could unite our bodies and psyches to the authentic Self. Without becoming rude and rough to keep healthy, we could learn to give life to the little barbarians in us. Maybe, in this process of discovering our authentic Selves, we can help to avoid and heal depression, anxiety, and other forms of isolation.

Science can benefit from the study of traditional forms of healing. Research about the healing effect of the voice has revealed for example, that cultivated forms of intensive singing increases the immune globulin level, improving the immune system of the body. Singing daily could be seen as a simple form of health insurance. The anticipation of relief or improvement of pain or distress can trigger our mind-body connection and can help deal with health issues. Modern scientists like Dr. Alvord have experienced the amazing impacts of non-pharmacological and non-medical forms of healing on patients.

Not only traditional singing helps in the process of healing. In a recent study of patients with Parkinson's disease–a neurological disorder causing a failure to produce dopamine–a, placebo injection of a neurotransmitter caused a real chemical change. The brain scan on those patients confirmed that the causative factor in the healing effect was their belief in the reduction of distress, which produced dopamine. Sham medication, injections and even pretend surgery can stimulate the power of suggestion to heal the body. Similar to this effect, belief in cultural rituals, trustworthy forms of treatment with authentic contact, can stimulate chemical responses with real effects of healing.

The voice as therapeuticum is an instrument for self-healing, also vibrating and connecting body and mind. Influencing blood pressure, heartbeat and the formatio reticularis, a network of the brain activating the limbic system, the voice can regulate emotions and primitive drives and instincts. Freeing up energy through the voice can also create–beside emotional, social and spiritual effects–chemical, physical and neurological changes.From the babble sound of infants, through primitive music such as Kurdish improvisations, Native Americans singing for survival, Islamite sing-reading, Greek sing-crying of laments, Indian and European virtuosity, bel canto, perfected opera, and pop music, to the treasured client experiences of my work, the therapeutic aspect is the human to human contact made through the human voice. Therapists and clients are not the only ones who need these relationships for professional and individual development. Through the essential tool of authentic voice and authentic singing, anyone and everyone can finally reclaim and enjoy the healing power of authentic human contact.

LAUGH

BECAUSE THAT IS THE PUREST

SOUND

INFORMATION ABOUT VOICE WORKSHOPS AND MUSIC THERAPY

WORKSHOPS:

"A Time To Sing", "Singing a Personal and Professional Need" or other voice training: www.TouchingVoices.com; TouchingVoices@yahoo.com;

MUSIC THERAPY:

AMTA American Music Therapy Association; www.musictherapy.org;

World Federation of Music Therapy, Incorporated (WFMT): www.musictherapyworld.net; www.voices.no;

European Consortium for Arts Therapies Education: www.ecarte.info;

<u>Contact</u>: Kate Richards Geller: Singforyourself@yahoo.com

Sylka Uhlig: Sylka.Uhlig@han.nl; or at: HAN Hogeschool Arnhem / Nijmegen (University for Professional education), The Netherlands.

References

Adamek, K. (1996). Singen als Lebenshilfe, Zu Empirie und Theorie von Alltagsbewältigungen, Plädoyer für eine erneute Kultur des Singens. Münster/New York: Waxmann Verlag.

Aldridge, D. (2005). Music therapy and neurological rehabilitation. (Ed.) London and Philadelphia: Jessica Kingsley Publishers.

Allegri, Renzo and Roberto (1997). Callas by Callas, The secret writings of Ala Maria. Milan: Arnoldo Mondadori Editore S.p.A., Artes Graficas Toledo, S.A.

Allen, Ware & Garrison (1867). Slave songs of the United States. Bedford, Massachusetts: Applewood Books.

Alvarez, A. & Reid, S, (1999). Autism and personality: Findings from the Tavistock autism workshop. London and New York: Routledge Taylor & Francis Group.

Alvord, Arviso Lori, M.D. & Cohen van Pelt, Elizabeth (2000). The Scalpel and the silver bear: the first Navajo woman surgeon combines western medicine and traditional healing. New York, Toronto, London, Sydney, Auckland: Bantam Books, Random House.

Andrews, T. (1993) Animal speak, the spiritual & magical power of creatures great & small. St. Paul Minnesota, USA: Llewellyn Publications A Division of Llewellyn Worldwide.

Andrews, T. (1996). Sacred sound, transformation through music & word. St. Paul, Minnesota, USA: Llewellyn Publications.

Ansdell, G. (1995). Music for life: Aspects of creative music therapy with adult clients. London: Jessica Kingsley Publishers.

Austin, D. (1993). Projection of parts of the self onto music and musical instrument. In Your inner music, creative analysis and music memory by Rolla M.R. Wilmette, Illinois: Chiron Publications.

Austin, D. (1998). When the psyche sings: Transference and countertransference, improvised singing with individual adults. In Dynamics of music psychotherapy by Bruscia (Ed.). Gilsum, NH: Barcelona Publishers.

Austin, D. (1999). Many stories, many songs. In Inside music therapy, client experiences by Hibben, J. (Ed.). Gilsum, NH: Barcelona Publishers.

Austin, D. (1999). Vocal improvisation in analytical oriented music therapy with adults. In Clinical Applications of music therapy in psychiatry by Wilgram, T & Bakker, De, J. (Eds.). (p. 141-155). London and Philadelphia: Jessica Kingsley Publishers.

Baumann, M. (2004). Wo steht die Musiktherapie in der Neurorehabilitation? In Musiktherapeutische Umschau, Band 25 2004, 1. Göttingen, Germany: Vandenhoeck & Ruprecht.
Beaulieu, J. (1987). Music and sound in the healing arts. New York: Station Hill Press.
Behrendt, J. E. (1990). Ik hoor - dus ik ben, werkboek & leesboek over de kunst van het luisteren. Katwijk, The Netherlands: Panta Rhei.
Behrendt, J. E. (1992). Das dritte Ohr, vom Hören der Welt. Hamburg, Germany: Rowohlt Taschenbuch Verlag GmbH.
Berger, D. (2002). Music therapy, sensory integration and the autistic child. London and Philadelphia: Jessica Kingsley Publishers.
Blum, S./Hassanpour, A. (1996). Popular music, Vol. 15, No.3, Middle East Issue (Oct.,1996), 325-343. www.jstor.org.
Blumenfeld L. (Ed.) (1993). Book and CD's. Voices of forgotten worlds: Traditional music of in indigenous people. Roslyn, New York: Ellipsis arts. Produced in Cooperation with the United Nations Centre For Human Rights.
Bossinger, W. (2005). Die Heilende Kraft des Singens. Norderstedt, Germany, Books on Demand GmbH.
Botani, B. (1991). Heyranok Gili u gazinden evine Muzik u mork. Spanga Sweden: Wesanxaneya Apec-Förlag Utgivare.
Briggs, C. A. (1991). A model for understanding musical development. In Music Therapy, vol. 10, No. 1, 1-21.
Bruscia, K. (1991). Case studies in music therapy. Phoenixville: Barcelona Publishers.
Buber, Martin (1947, 1975, 1991). Tales of the Hasidim. New York: Schocken Books Inc. Amazon.com.
Choksy, J.K. (1998). Purity and pollution in Zoroastrianism, triumph over evil. Austin: University of Texas Press.
Christensen, D. (1975). On Variability in Kurdish Dance Songs. In Asian Music, Vol. 6 No.1/2, Perspectives on Asian Music: Essays in Honor of Dr. Laurence E. R. Picken (1975), 1-6. www.jstor.org.
Collins, S.K. & Kuck, K. (1991). Music therapy in the neonatal intensive care unit. In Neonatal Network, Vol. 9 No.6.
Cook, P. M. (1997). Book and CD. Shaman, Jhankri & Nele, Music healers of indigenous cultures. New York: Ellipsis Art.
Crabtree, A. (1999). Trance Zero, The psychology of maximum experience. New York: St. Martin's Press.
Cramer, A. (1998). Das Buch von der Stimme, Ihre formende und heilende Kraft verstehen und erfahren. Zürich/Düsseldorf, Germany: Walter Verlag.

Dame, J. (1994). Het zingend lichaam, betekenissen van de stem in Westerse vocale muziek. Proefschrift Universiteit van Amsterdam, The Netherlands: Kok Agora, Kampen.

Dekker-Voigt, H.H. & Knill, P. J. & Weymann, E. (1996). Lexikon Musiktherapie. Göttingen, Bern, Toronto, Seattle: Hogrefe-Verlag.

Dethlefsen T. & Dahlke, R. (1989). Krankheit als Weg, Deutung and Be-Deutung der Krankheitsbilder. München, Germany: Wilhelm Goldmann Verlag.

Dileo, C. (Ed.) (1999). Music therapy & medicine: Theoretical and clinical applications. Silver Spring, MD: American Music Therapy Association.

During, Jean (1994). Kurdistan, Zikr et chants soufis. CD cover Radio France ocora.

Everett, S. (1999). History of Slavery. New Jersey: Chartwell Books Inc.

Flatscher, R. (1992). The forgotten power of rhythm. Mendocino, CA: LifeRhythm.

Frohne, I. (1981). Das Rhythmische Prinzip, Grundlagen, Formen und Realisationsbeispiele in Therapie und Pädagogik. Germany: Eres Edition.

Gaynor, M. M.D. (2002). The Healing power of sound, recovery from life-threatening illness using sound, voice and music. Boston & London: Shambhala.

Ghiglieri, Michael P. (1999). The dark side of man. tracing the origins of male violence. Reading, Massachusetts: Perseus Books

Gladwell, M. (2005). Blink, the power of thinking without thinking. New York, Boston: Little, Brown and Company.

Goleman, D. (1998). Working with emotional intelligence. New York: Bantam Books.

Gunter, M. M. (1990). The Kurds in Turkey, a political dilemma. Westview special studies on the Middle East, Colorado: Westview Press.

Gustorff, D. & Hannich H-J. (2000). Jenseits des Wortes, Musiktherapie mit komatösen Patienten auf der Intersivstation. Bern, Göttingen, Toronto, Saettle, Germany: Verlag Hans Huber.

Güvenç. O. (...). Orientalische Musik - und Kunsttherapie, Der orientalische Ansatz Krankheiten mit künstlerischen Medien zu heilen & ihr heutiger Stand. Rosenau, Austria: Schule für Altorientalische Musik und Kunsttherapie.

Hafiz, (1999). The Gift, poems by Hafiz the great Sufi master. New York: ARKANA, Penguin Books.

Hamel, P. M. (1986). Durch Musik zum Selbst, Wie man Musik neu erleben und erfahren kann. Germany, München: Deutscher Taschenbuch Verlag. Kassel, Basel, London: Bärenreiter-Verlag.

Hegi, F. (1988). Improvisation und Musiktherapie, Möglichkeiten und Wirkungen von freier Musik. Paderborn, Germany: Jungfermann Verlag.

Hewitt, G. (1981). How To Sing. London: EMI Music Publishing Ltd.

Holst-Warhaft, G. (1992). Dangerous voices, women's laments and Greek literature. London and New York: Routledge.

Institut Kurde (1989). CD cover: Sivan Perwer chants du Kurdistan. Made in France: Institut Kurde, 106 Rue La Fayette, 75010 Paris.

Janov, A. (1972). The primal scream, primal therapy: The cure of neurosis: New York: Dell Publishing Co., Inc.

Jourdain, R. (2001). Das wohltemperierte Gehirn, Wie Musik im Kopf entsteht und wirkt. Germany, Heidelberg, Berlin: Spektrum Akademischer Verlag.

Jung, C. G. (1964). Man and his symbols. New York: Anchor Books, Doubleday, J. G. Ferguson Publishing.

Jung, C. G. (1974). Dreams. New York: MJF Books, Fine Communications by Princeton University Press.

Karolyi, O. (1998). Traditional African & Oriental music. Harmondsworth, Middlesex, England: Penguin books.

Keeney, Bradford, Ph.D. (Ed.) (2001). Walking Thunder: Dine Medicine Woman, Profiles of Healing. Philadelphia: Ringing Rocks Press.

Kovach, A. M. S. (1985). Shamanism and guided imagery and music: A comparison. Journal of Music Therapy, XXII (3), 1985, 154-165.

Laizer, S. (1991). Into Kurdistan, frontiers under fire. London and New Jersey: Zed Books Ltd.

Larousse, H. G. (Ed.) (1971). The Larousse encyclopedia of music. New York: Crescent Books, Crown Publishers.

Lessac, A. (1967). The use and training of the human voice: A practical approach to speech and voice dynamics. Mountain View, California: Mayfield Publishing Company.

Loewy, J. V. (1995). The musical stages of speech: a developmental model of pre-verbal sound making. In Music Therapy, 1995, Vol.13, No. 1, 47-73.

Loewy, J. V. (2004). Integrating music, language and voice in music therapy; VOICES: Main Issues Vol.4 no.1, Art#140, March 1, 2004.

McCullough-Brabson, Ellen & Help, Marilyn (2001). We'll be in your mountains, we'll be in your songs, a Navajo woman sings. University of New Mexico Press.

Michels, U. (Ed.) (1985). dtv-Atlas zur Musik, Tafeln und Texte. Deutscher Taschenbuch Verlag, Germany: Bärenreiter Verlag.

Monk, M. (2000). Stagebill, Lincoln Center Festival, New York.

Montello, L. (2002). Essential musical intelligence, using music as your path to healing, creativity, and radiant wholeness. Quest Books, Theosophical Publishing House Wheaton, Illinois, Chennai (Madras), India.

Moses, P. (1954). The voice of neurosis. New York, San Francisco, London: Grune & Stratton.

Nakkach, S. Vox Mundi Project USA. (1999/2005). The yoga of the voice snakkach@cs.com / voxmundiproject.com / voxmundi@yahoo.com.

Newham, P. (1998). Therapeutic voicework, principles and practice for the use of singing as a therapy. London and Philadelphia: Jessica Kingsley Publishers.

Nöcker-Ribaupierre, M. (2003). Hören–Brücke ins Leben. Musiktherapie mit früh- und neugeborenen Kindern. Göttingen, Germany: Vandenhoeck & Ruprecht.

Nordoff, P. & Robbins, C. (1977). Creative music therapy, Individualized treatment for the handicapped child. John Day & Co: New York.

O'Kane, F. (1994). Sacred chaos, reflections on God's shadow and the dark self. Toronto, Canada: Inner City Books.

Poché, C. (1974/1989). CD cover: Kurdish music musique Kurde. Made in France: Conseil International De La Musique. AUVIDIS-UNESCO.

Rashid, Xalid (1996). CD cover: Musique du Kurdistan, music from Kurdistan. Made in France: Music from the world. CD 92668-2.

Razbar Ensemble (2002)). Leyli, Iran-chants sacres Kurdes. CD cover Disques ARION, Made in France, ARN 64576.

Richards Geller, K. (1997). The voice of pain: The use of the voice in music therapy with hospitalized children undergoing intrusive medical procedures. New York: Unpublished master thesis.

Rosenberg, D. (1999). CD cover: The Gypsy road–a musical migration from India to Spain. Durham, NC 27715-2043, USA: Alula Records.

Sacks, O. (1985). The man who mistook his wife for a hat; and other clinical tales. New York: Summit Books.

Scheiby, B. (1998). The role of musical countertransference in analytical music therapy. In dynamics of music psychotherapy by Bruscia (Ed.). Gilsum, NH: Barcelona Publishers.

Schwarts & Ritchie (1999). Music listening in neonatal intensive care units. In Dileo, C. (Ed.) Music therapy & medicine: Theoretical and clinical applications. Silver Spring, MD: American Music Therapy Association.

Smeijsers, H. (1991). Muziektherapie als psychotherapy. Assen/Maastricht, The Netherlands: Van Gorcum.

Sokolov, L. (1981). The therapeutic process of finding one's voice. New York: Unpublished manuscript.

Spitzer, M. (2003). Musik im Kopf, Hören, Musizieren, Verstehen und Erleben im Neuronalen Netxwerk. Stuttgart, New York: Schattauer.

Standley, M. J. (1991). The role of music in pacification/stimulation of premature infants with low birthweights. Florida State University: Center for Music Research.

Standley, M. J. (2003). Music therapy with premature infants, research and developmental interventions, Silver Spring, MD: The American Music Therapy Association

Stein, J. (1966). The Random House dictionary of the English language. New York: Random House.

Storms, G. (1985). Muziek en dans uit India, kennismaking met een fascinerende muziekcultuur. Katwijk aan Zee, The Netherlands: Servire Uitgever.

Temo, Nasir&Bedirxan (1995). Kurdish songs and music, CD cover CD B 6815 AUVDIS ETHNIC.

VPRO (1999). Dutch television program in 7 parts "Lied van verdriet", videos. The Netherlands: VPRO Publieksservice, Postbus 11, 1200 JC Hilversum.

Watzlawick, P. (1978). Wie wirklich ist die Wirklichkeit? Wahn Täuschung Verstehen. München, Germany: R. Piper & Co Verlag.

Wilber, K. (1996). A brief history of everything. Boston & London: Shambhala.

Suggested Reading

Austin, D. (1993). Projection of parts of the self onto music and musical instrument, in *Your Inner Music, Creative Analysis and Music Memory* by Rolla, M.R.Wilmette, Illinois: Chiron Publications.

Austin, D. (1999). Many stories, many songs. In *Inside musictherapy, client experiences* by Hibben, J. (Ed.). Lower Village, Gilsum, NH: Barcelona Publishers.

Baumann, M. (2004). Wo steht die Musiktherapie in der Neurorehabilitation? In *Musiktherapeutische Umschau*, Band 25 2004, 1,Vanderhoeck & Ruprecht, Göttingen.

Behrendt, J. E. (1990). *Ik hoor - dus ik ben, werkboek & leesboek over de kunst van het luisteren*. Katwijk, The Netherlands: Panta Rhei.

Behrendt, J. E. (1992). *Das dritte Ohr, vom Hören der Welt.* Hamburg, Germany: Rowohlt Taschenbuch Verlag GmbH.

Blum, S./Hassanpour, A. (1996). *Popular music*, Vol. 15, No.3, Middle East Issue (Oct.,1996), 325-343. www.jstor.org.

Botani, B. (1991). *Heyranok Gili u gazinden evine Muzik u mork.* Spanga Sweden: Wesanxaneya Apec-Förlag Utgivare.

Bruscia, K. (1991). *Case studies in music therapy.* Phoenixville: Barcelona Publishers.

Choksy, J.K. (1998). *Purity and pollution in Zoroastrianism, triumph over evil.* Austin: University of Texas Press.

Christensen, D. (1975). On variability in Kurdish dance songs. In *Asian Music*, Vol. 6 No.1/2, Perspectives on Asian Music: Essays in Honor of Dr. Laurence E. R. Picken (1975), 1-6. www.jstor.org.

Dame, J.(1994). *Het zingend lichaam, betekenissen van de stem in Westerse vocale muziek.* Proefschrift Universiteit van Amsterdam, The Netherlands: Kok Agora, Kampen.

Dethlefsen T. & Dahlke, R. (1989). *Krankheit als Weg, Deutung and Be-Deutung der Krankheitsbilder.* München, Germany: Wilhelm Goldmann Verlag.

Dileo, C. (Ed.) (1999). *Music therapy & medicine: Theoretical and clinical applications.* Silver Spring, MD: American Music Therapy Association.

Everett, S. (1999). History of slavery. New Jersey: Chartwell Books Inc.

Flatscher, R. (1992). *The forgotten power of rhythm.* Mendocino, CA: LifeRhythm.

Frohne, I. (1981). *Das Rhythmische Prinzip, Grundlagen, Formen und Realisationsbeispiele in Therapie und Pädagogik.* Germany: Eres Edition.
Goleman, D. (1998). *Working with emotional intelligence.* New York: Bantam Books.
Gunter, M. M. (1990) *The Kurds in Turkey, A political dilemma.* Westview special studies on the Middle East, Colorado: Westview Press.
Hamel, P. M. (1986). *Durch Musik zum Selbst, Wie man Musik neu erleben und erfahren kann.* Germany, München: Deutscher Taschenbuch Verlag. Kassel, Basel, London: Bärenreiter-Verlag.
Hewitt, G. (1981). *How to sing.* London: EMI Music Publishing Ltd.
Jourdain, R. (2001). *Das wohltemperierte Gehirn, Wie Musik im Kopf entsteht und wirkt.* Germany, Heidelberg, Berlin: Spektrum Akademischer Verlag.
Jung, C. G. (1974). *Dreams.* New York: MJF Books, Fine Communications by Princeton University Press.
Linklater, C. (1976). *Freeing the natural voice.* New York: Drama publishers.
Michels, U. (Ed.)(1985). *dtv-Atlas zur Musik,* Tafeln und Texte. Deutscher Taschenbuch Verlag, Germany: Bärenreiter Verlag.
Sacks, O. (1985). *The man who mistook his wife for a hat; and other clinical tales.* New York: Summit Books.
Spitzer, M. (2003) *Musik im Kopf, Hören, Musizieren, Verstehen und Erleben im Neuronalen Netzwerk.* Stuttgart, New York: Schattauer.
VPRO (1999). Dutch television program in 7 parts *"Lied van verdriet,"* videos. The Netherlands: VPRO Publieksservice, Postbus 11, 1200 JC Hilversum.
Watzlawick, P. (1978). *Wie wirklich ist die Wirklichkeit? Wahn Täuschung Verstehen,* München, Germany: R. Piper & Co Verlag.

Appendix C

Kurdish Scales (Maqams)

Some of these are also used in Arabic and Islamic music. (Botani, 1991, p. 16) Musical signs for microtones in Arabic and Islamic music are as follows. (Karolyi, 1998, p.67-68):

♯ = sharp ; 𝄲 = half sharp ; 𝄰 = 3/4 sharp ; ♭ = flat ; 𝄳 or 𝄳 = half flat ; 𝄫 = 3/4 flat

Beyat kurdî

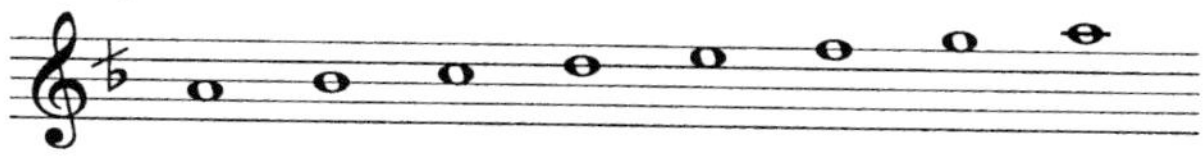

Hicaz kurdî

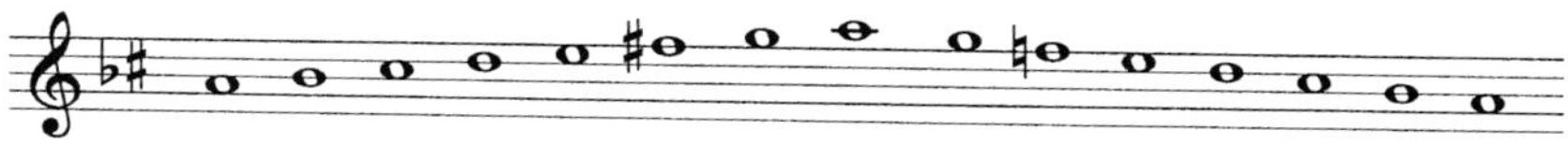

Kurd

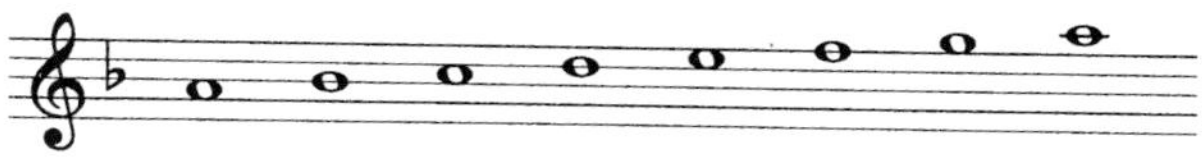

Nehawend

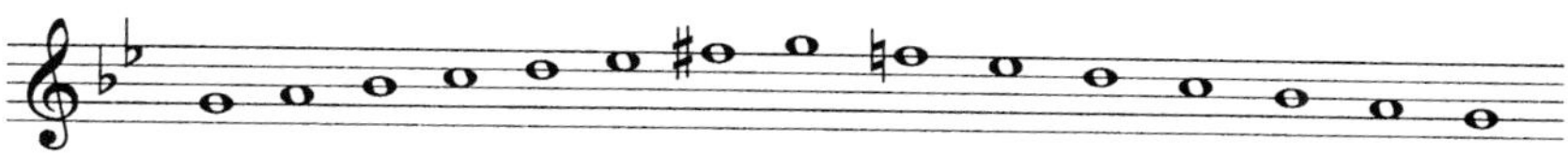

Ecem

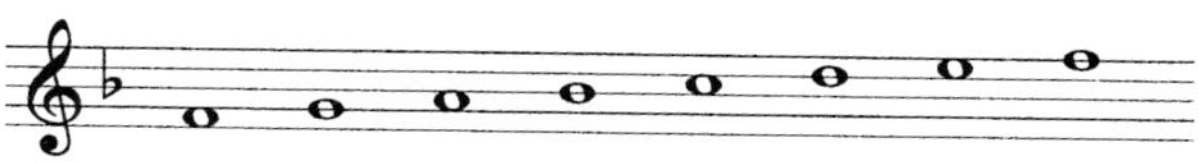

Rast

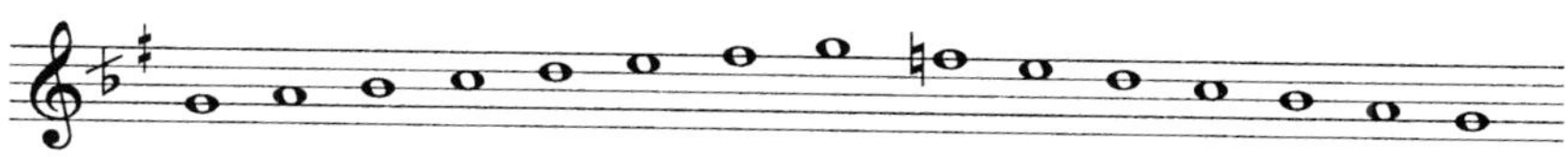

Seba

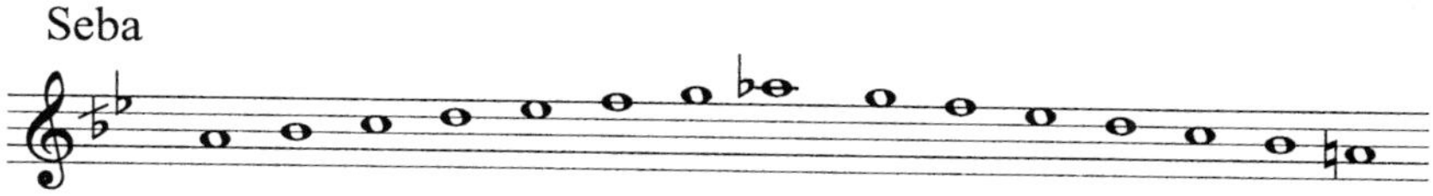

Sêgeh

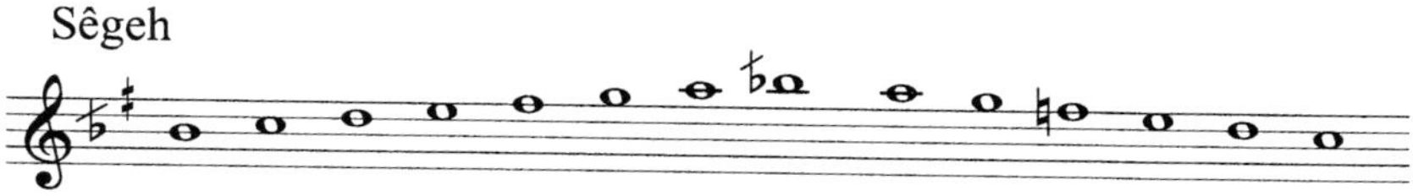

Appendix B: Indigenous Songs

In the collection of *Voices of Forgotten Worlds*, edited by Blumenfeld and made with support of the United Nations Centre For Human Rights, I found more treasures of primitive songs. It is a powerful collection of political, environmental, individual and cultural voices with many comments by original musicians. The "indigenous people are the original inhabitants of the lands that have been colonized or overrun by others. . . . Indigenous peoples have been called the guardians of the earth. . . . [They] are also the caretakers of cultures, customs, philosophies and ways of life" (Burger in Blumenfeld, p. 5).

Tuva. The shamans from Tuva, in the south of Siberia, have recently revitalized their tradition after an interruption from the Communist Soviet regime. "Every Tuvan Shaman has his own helping animal spirits. With his voice he may call on aid from these animals or make other animal sounds that are used for specific purpose. A cuckoo call to quiet a child, a raven's crow to scare away bad people and an owl's hoot to calm the cattle" (Cook, 1997, p. 46). The Tuvan shamans are renowned for their throat singing where one singer produces two notes simultaneously. The bottom note, a kind of drone serves as the fundamental tone. The whistling sounds heard are the overtones, or harmonics, of that same tone. The varieties of tones made through these different combinations are endless and create exceptional effects. Professor Ted Levin writes,

> "Tuvan throat-singing is most of all a meditation on a place, on spirits that inhabit that place, and on ancestors that once inhabited it. It changes the way you listen." (Levin in Blumenfeld, p. 15)

Pygmy. In the rainforest of Central Africa live the Pygmies, the largest population of hunter-gatherers and the shortest human beings. "The name 'Pygmy' dates back to ancient Greece, although Pygmies appear in the historical record long before that time. After Aristotle, however, the Pygmies were considered to be a myth. . . . The Pygmies' musical ceremonies are magnificent. The art of the *mokoondi*, a social assembly where 'the jungle spirits and the low yodeling of the women' . . . 'chant into the night', impress, invite and influence the whole community. As usual the women's voices create a spiritual meeting at one end of the camp when they start to sing. Everyone around, men and boys, utter their high-pitched cries. The ceremony continues with ritualistic walking of men along a path into the forest. The vocal noise changes into a 'chorus of two-note cries approached' and 'the women set off in pursuit, dancing after it. 'YO!' everyone cried." (Sarno in Blumenfeld, p. 66)

Australia. In the Aboriginal tradition, was it vital to 'sing the world into existence' as help for daily survival. Aboriginal creation myths tell of famous totemic beings who wandered over the Australian continent in the 'dreamtime,' singing out the name of everything that crossed their path–births, animals, plants, rocks–in a sense, singing the world into existence. 'Dreaming tracks,' or *'songlines'* to the Australian Aboriginal people, are 'the footprints of the ancestors' or 'way of the law,' the core of an intricate connection between everyday life, ancestry and natural surroundings. They serve as the key to an existence that fuses the everyday with the timeless, the ordinary world with the spiritual world. A song was both map and direction finder. Given that you know the song, you always were able to find your way across the country. And a man on 'walkabout' would always be traveling down one of the *songlines.* In these old days there were no other ways to find the directions.

> 'Suppose the man strayed from his *Songline*?' 'He was trespassing–he might get speared for it.' 'But as long as he stuck to the track he'd always find people who shared his dreaming? Who were his brothers?' 'Yes.' (Bruce Chatwin, in Blumenfeld, p. 34)

Inuits (Eskimos). The Inuit people live throughout Greenland, Northern Canada, Alaska and parts of Siberia and share a strong singing tradition. "*Inngerutit*, their drum-song tradition, was once an integral part of their lives. Not only did Inuit people sing at feasts, they sang every day–when they were out sealing, when they were at home, when they felt sorrow, anger or joy."

The drum-song style of the Inuits shows similarities to shamanistic singing where the whole body of the singer is involved: "He begins to sing a melodic chant over the beat as he turns his body left, and then right. Bending at the knees, he springs up again and again, moving the drum side-to-side, completely absorbed in his drum-song." (Blumenfeld, p. 42)

The traditional Inuit musical forms span a wide range of vocal, glottal sounds formed in the throat, and verbal agglutinations[70], literary gluing words together. Some of the song styles follow: "*Anarsaatit* expresses moods and feelings, often with beautiful allusions to nature. *Aqaatit* sing of sealing and the hunt. *Mumerit* involve role-playing games."

---

70. Agglutination: the formation of words by adding separate constituents, each with a distinct meaning.

Especially interesting are the duel-songs, called *pisit*, where two singers are pitted against each other, often to resolve social problems. Standing face to face, they produce piquant sounds and the audience is asked to pick the winner. (pp. 44)[71]

New Zealand. The Maori people, known as the warrior race of New Zealand, "have been tied to their land ever since with a fierce determination." The Traditional music of the Maori contains 'action songs' and chants. Action songs are performed with interesting hand gestures and a form of sign language. *Waiata* and *Haka* are the two traditional styles of chants. *Waiata* are mainly common and nowadays are used in welcome ceremonies. *Haka* are war dances. These originate from their great battles and were intriguingly performed to insult or 'scare off' enemies. To impress their enemies they would utter their dangerous expressions bodily and vocally: "Opposing armies would stand 200 meters apart and, while they chanted, they would stick their tongues out, roll their eyes, grimace and snarl." (Te Rangi Huata in Blumenfeld, p. 5)

Tibetan. The Ladakhi share Tibetan Buddhist culture, religion and language. In one of the driest and highest inhabited regions in the world, where the land is frozen eight months of the year, and when fields are surrounded by areas of rock and desert, the people of Ladakh prosper. "[W]hat the Ladakhis have had for centuries [is] the balance with the natural world and the essential harmony in terms of relationships. . . . In summer, the Ladakhis take advantage of the warm weather to throw lots of parties. The first requirement for a party is a nice garden, which is really something special in this arid country . . . musicians play . . . and everybody dances. There's always a popular local sport . . . even the monks join in these diversions. Wherever Ladakhis are hard at work–in the fields, carrying loads in the street, building houses–they sing work songs. The leader sings a brief phrase, and the others respond, as simple as, 'Now we are cutting the grain,' or 'Now this plot is cleared.' They exhibit an incredible joy in life." (Lewiston in Blumenfeld, p. 61)

Japan. The Ainu people, whose name means 'man,' live in northern island of Japan and were the original hunting-gathering population, in stark contrast to the Japanese, Koreans and Chinese, who had been agriculturists. "Ainu religion is a mixture of shamanism and animism. Deities are believed to appear to the Ainu in disguise, often in the form of animals. For example, a bear, worshiped above all animals, is seen as the mountain deity bringing gifts of meat and hide. . . . Although the Ainu express their religious beliefs in daily ritual, they are best articulated through their oral tradition, which contains many genres. Epic or lyric verses are sung or chanted, and narrative prose is recited. . .

---

71. In the movie *The Long Runner*, made by an Inuit in traditional language and with exotic rituals, some of these traditions are shown.

. Most songs carry melodies that consist only of two or three different notes. Many include mimicry of animal cries and birds singing." (Michel in Blumenfeld, p. 18)

India. The Indian tradition of healing is well known and the singing voice is important for the celebration of mantras. A mantra is a sacred word or the name of a god, "contained in chant-like melodies, repetitive rhythms and changing vocal dynamics . . . [and] dramatic exaggerated in-breaths." The patient is "coaxed through sing-song dialogues to identify his or her illness," as explained by an Indian shaman about shamanic healing music. "The ghost blocks the voice" of the patient, "the body shakes wildly; even his head hits the floor and turns quickly from side to side. This is the ghost resisting my treatment." (Cook, 1997, p. 11)

Appendix C: Vibration of Human Vowel

Picture of the vibration of a human vowel[72] (Cramer, 1998, p. 231):

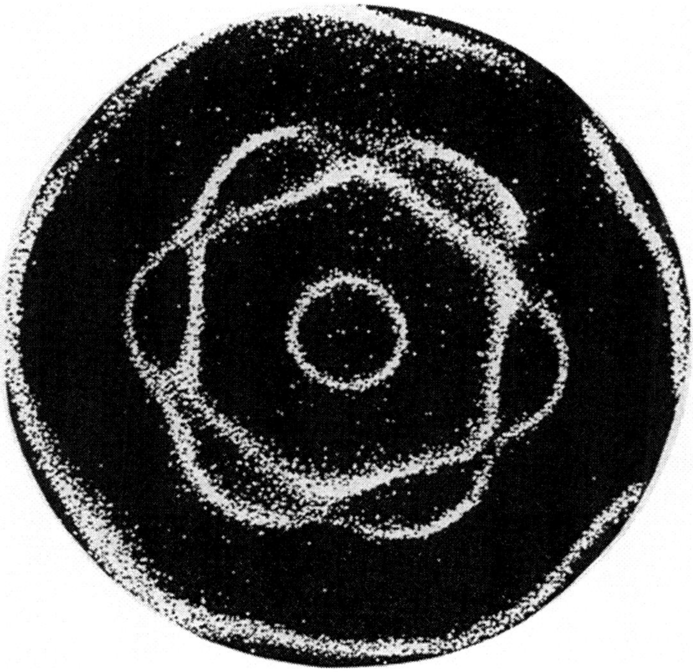

72 "In 1967, the late Hans Jenny, a Swiss doctor, artist, and researcher, published the bilingual book Kymatik -Wellen und Schwingungen mit ihrer Struktur und Dynamik/ Cymatics - The Structure and Dynamics of Waves and Vibrations. In this book Jenny, like Chladni two hundred years earlier, showed what happens when one takes various materials like sand, spores, iron filings, water, and viscous substances, and places them on vibrating metal plates and membranes. Jenny made use of crystal oscillators and an invention of his own by the name of the tonoscope to set these plates and membranes vibrating. This was a major step forward. The advantage with crystal oscillators is that one can determine exactly which frequency and amplitude/volume one wants. It was now possible to research and follow a continuous train of events in which one had the possibility of changing the frequency or the amplitude or both. The tonoscope was constructed to make the human voice visible without any electronic apparatus as an intermediate link. This yielded the amazing possibility of being able to see the physical image of the vowel, tone or song a human being produced directly. Not only could you hear a melody - you could see it, too!" (Peter Pettersson. 2002-2006. http://www.world-mysteries.com).